Radiology

CLINICAL CASES UNCOVERED

Ashley S. Shaw
MB ChB, MRCP, FRCR
Department of Radiology
Addenbrooke's Hospital
Cambridge, UK

Edmund M. Godfrey
BM BCh, MA, MRCS
Department of Radiology
Addenbrooke's Hospital
Cambridge, UK

Abhinav Singh
BSc, MBBS, MRCS
Department of Radiology
Addenbrooke's Hospital
Cambridge, UK

Tarik F. Massoud
MA, MD, PhD, FRCR
Department of Radiology
Addenbrooke's Hospital and University of Cambridge
Cambridge, UK

WILEY-BLACKWELL
A John Wiley & Sons, Ltd., Publication

Blackwell Publishing was acquired by John Wiley & Sons in February 2007. Blackwell's publishing program has been merged with Wiley's global Scientific, Technical and Medical business to form Wiley-Blackwell.

Registered office: John Wiley & Sons Ltd, The Atrium, Southern Gate, Chichester, West Sussex, PO19 8SQ, UK

Editorial offices: 9600 Garsington Road, Oxford, OX4 2DQ, UK
　　　　　　　　The Atrium, Southern Gate, Chichester, West Sussex, PO19 8SQ, UK
　　　　　　　　111 River Street, Hoboken, NJ 07030-5774, USA

For details of our global editorial offices, for customer services and for information about how to apply for permission to reuse the copyright material in this book please see our website at www.wiley.com/wiley-blackwell

Library of Congress Cataloging-in-Publication Data

Radiology / Ashley Shaw ... [et al.].
　　p. ; cm. – (Clinical cases uncovered)
　Includes indexes.
　ISBN 978-1-4051-8474-8
　1. Radiography, Medical–Case studies.　I. Shaw, Ashley, Dr.　II. Series: Clinical cases uncovered.
　[DNLM:　1. Radiography–methods–Case Reports.　WN 180 R1288 2009]
　RC78.15.R276 2009
　616.07′572–dc22

　　　　　　　　　　　　　　　　　　　　　　　　　　　　　　　　2009004427

ISBN: 9781405184748

A catalogue record for this book is available from the British Library.

Set in 9/12 pt Minion by SNP Best-set Typesetter Ltd., Hong Kong
Printed and bound in Singapore by Ho Printing Singapore Pte Ltd

1　2009

Contents

Colour plate section can be found facing p. 54.

Preface

Radiology, unlike many other specialties in medicine, cannot be studied in isolation. In determining what investigation is most appropriate, one needs to appreciate what the clinical problem is, what the potential causes are and what other comorbidities the patient has. To interpret an investigation, one needs to understand anatomy, physiology and pathology. Technological advances in radiology over the past decades have revolutionized the management of patients in all branches of medicine. Many medical and surgical specialties rely upon the radiologist to make the diagnosis, assess response to therapy and identify any complications that may arise.

This textbook is divided in to three sections. The first section gives the core information for the reader to understand radiological principles, with an explanation of common terminology and techniques, the use of contrast media within radiology and the risks associated with ionizing radiation. The second part of the book is devoted to clinical cases. In reading through these, the reader will be set a clinical scenario and be challenged in how they might investigate such a case, their interpretation of clinical and radiological findings and their management of these findings. The cases vary in difficulty and style according to the conditions being discussed, but the case-based question and answer scheme is constant. At the end of each case, there is a review and a summary of the key points. The final section is for self-assessment: 30 multiple choice questions, 10 structured answer questions and 10 extended matching questions all designed to test the reader's understanding of radiology and, more importantly, its applications in a range of clinical scenarios.

The purpose of this book is not to make the reader in to a competent radiologist or to simply supply them with a list of facts and differential diagnoses. The aim is to engage the reader in real-life clinical scenarios, to begin to understand how and when to investigate patients, and to develop an approach to looking at radiological images. Furthermore, this book will serve as a review of many commonly encountered conditions and their radiological appearances.

Ashley S. Shaw
Edmund M. Godfrey
Abhinav Singh
Tarik F. Massoud

Acknowledgements

We, the authors, would like to acknowledge our colleagues within the Department of Radiology at Addenbrooke's Hospital, Cambridge who helped us to compile the images for this book: Helen Addley, Owen Arthurs, Judith Babar, Sue Barter, Nicholas Carroll, H. K. Cheow Justin Cross, Alan Freeman, Brendan Koo, Anant Krishnan, Evis Sala, Daniel Scoffings, Teik Choon See, Patricia Set, Ruchi Sinnatamby and Nagui Antoun.

We wish to extend our thanks to Julian Evans, for his assistance in preparing the images, and to the radiology staff at Addenbrooke's Hospital, Cambridge for all their help during the preparation of this book.

Finally, we wish to show our appreciation for the help and guidance of Laura Murphy, Ben Townsend and the staff at Wiley-Blackwell for all their assistance in the production of the book, from conception to publication.

How to use this book

Clinical Cases Uncovered (CCU) books are carefully designed to help supplement your clinical experience and assist with refreshing your memory when revising. Each book is divided in to three sections: Part 1, Basics; Part 2, Cases; and Part 3, Self-Assessment.

Part 1 gives a quick reminder of the basic science, history and examination, and key diagnoses in the area. Part 2 contains many of the clinical presentations you would expect to see on the wards or crop up in exams, with questions and answers leading you through each case. New information, such as test results, is revealed as events unfold and each case concludes with a handy case summary explaining the key points. Part 3 allows you to test your learning with several question styles (MCQs, EMQs and SAQs), each with a strong clinical focus.

Whether reading individually or working as part of a group, we hope you will enjoy using your CCU book. If you have any recommendations on how we could improve the series, please do let us know by contacting us at: medstudentuk@oxon.blackwellpublishing.com.

Disclaimer

CCU patients are designed to reflect real life, with their own reports of symptoms and concerns. Please note that all names used are entirely fictitious and any similarity to patients, alive or dead, is coincidental.

List of abbreviations

AAA	abdominal aortic aneurysm
AAST	American Association for the Surgery of Trauma
ADEM	acute disseminated encephalomyelitis
AFB	acid-fast bacilli
AFP	α-fetoprotein
ALL	acute lymphoblastic leukaemia
ALT	alanine aminotransferase
AML	angiomyolipoma
AP	antero-posterior
APACHE II	Acute Physiology and Chronic Health Evaluation Score II
APUD	amine precursor uptake and decarboxylase
AST	aspartate aminotransferase
ATLS	Advanced Trauma Life Support
BCG	bacille Calmette–Guérin
BTS	British Thoracic Society
CABG	coronary artery bypass graft
CLL	chronic lymphocytic leukaemia
CNS	central nervous system
COPD	chronic obstructive pulmonary disease
CR	complete response
CRP	C-reactive protein
CRu	complete response unconfirmed
CSF	cerebrospinal fluid
CT	computed tomography
CTPA	computed tomography pulmonary angiography/angiogram
DIP	distal interphalangeal
DLBCL	diffuse large B-cell lymphoma
DMARD	disease-modifying antirheumatic drug
DOTS	directly observed therapy
DSA	digital subtraction angiography/angiogram
EBV	Epstein–Barr virus
ECG	electrocardiogram
ERCP	endoscopic retrograde cholangiopancreatography
ESWL	extracorporeal shock wave lithotripsy
EVAR	endovascular aneurysm repair
FAST	focused assessment with sonography for trauma
FBC	full blood count
FDG-PET	2-[fluorine-18] fluoro-2-deoxy-D-glucose positron emission tomography
FNAC	fine needle aspiration cytology
GCS	Glasgow Coma Score
GGT	gamma glutamyl transferase
Hb	haemoglobin
HCC	hepatocellular carcinoma
HCG	human chorionic gonadotrophin
HDU	high dependency unit
HIDA	hepatobiliary imino-diacetic acid (scan)
HIFU	high intensity focused ultrasound
HRCT	high resolution computed tomography
HU	Hounsfield unit
HVA	homovanillic acid
ICP	intracranial presssure
Ig	immunoglobulin
INR	international normalized ratio
ITU	intensive therapy unit
IVP	intravenous pyelography
IVU	intravenous urography/urogram
KUB	kidney, ureter and bladder
LDH	lactate dehydrogenase
LFT	liver function test
MBP	myelin basic product
MCA	middle cerebral artery
MCV	mean cell volume
MDCT	multi-detector computed tomography
MHC	major histocompatibility complex
MIBG	metaiodobenzylguanidine
MRA	magnetic resonance angiography
MRCP	magnetic resonance cholangiopancreatography
MRI	magnetic resonance imaging
MS	multiple sclerosis

MTT	mean transit time	rCBV	regional cerebral blood volume
NHL	non-Hodgkin's lymphoma	RD	relapsed disease
NICE	National Institute for Clinical Excellence	RIND	reversible ischaemic neurological deficit
NSAID	non-steroidal anti-inflammatory drug	RRMS	relapsing remitting multiple sclerosis
NSLC	non-small cell lung cancer	SAH	subarachnoid haemorrhage
PA	postero–anterior	SD	stable disease
PACS	Patient Archiving and Communication Systems	SLE	systemic lupus erythematosus
PCNL	percutaneous nephrolithotomy	SPD	sum of the product of the greatest diameters
PCR	polymerase chain reaction	TB	tuberculosis
PD	progressive disease	TIA	transient ischaemic attack
PET	positron emission tomography	U+E	urea and electrolytes
Plt	platelets	VMA	vanillylmandelic acid
PPI	proton pump inhibitor	V/Q	ventilation–perfusion
PPMS	primary progressive multiple sclerosis	WCC	white cell count
PR	partial response	WFNS	World Federation of Neurological Surgeons
PT	prothrombin time		
rCBF	regional cerebral blood flow		

To my wife Abigail and children Beatrice and Jack. AS

To my wife Anna and my parents. EMG.

To my Mum, Dad and Sister Neha. AS.

To my children, Zahra and Adam. TFM.

Introduction to clinical radiology

Diagnostic imaging uses various forms of radiation (ionizing, e.g. X-rays, non-ionizing, e.g. soundwaves (ultrasound) and electromagnetic waves (MRI)) which interact with bodily tissues in a variety of ways to produce images which may yield anatomical and functional information. In contrast to these external sources of radiation, diagnostic nuclear medicine involves the administration of radioactive isotopes (usually orally or intravenously) which emit gamma-rays, or positrons, the distribution of which is imaged to give primarily functional information.

The X-ray

First discovered in 1895 by the German physicist Willhelm Conrad Röntgen, X-rays are high frequency electromagnetic waves that are produced by suddenly stopping fast-moving accelerated electrons at a metal target. As the X-rays pass through the body, they may be absorbed, scattered or transmitted, depending upon their interactions with the body tissues. The degree to which the X-ray beam is attenuated (absorbed or scattered) is dependent upon the energy of the X-rays and the effective atomic number of the tissues through which it passes. Hence, tissues with a higher effective atomic number (e.g. bone) will absorb more X-rays than those with a lower atomic number (e.g. air, soft tissues). Transmitted X-rays that reach and are absorbed by a detector (formerly a film) produce the radiograph (X-ray image).

Computed tomography

A computed tomography (CT) machine consists of two main components: the moving table on which the patient lies, and the gantry which houses the X-ray equipment and detectors, through which the table (and patient) move. When first introduced in to clinical practice in the 1970s, the X-ray tube moved around the patient in a step-and-shoot manner, taking several minutes to acquire each axial (transverse) image. Over the past three decades there have been many significant technological advances in CT technology. First, slip ring technology meant that the X-ray tube could continue to revolve around the patient (previously this was connected by electrical cables). With a fixed ring of detectors, the machine could acquire images continuously while the patient moved steadily through the gantry (hence spiral, or helical, CT). In recent years, manufacturers have replaced the single ring of detectors with multiple rows of detectors (multi-detector CT, MDCT), often now numbering in to the hundreds. These advances mean that the modern MDCT machine may acquire multiple contiguous slices, covering several centimetres, with each revolution of the X-ray tube (<0.5 s). Thus, the whole of the chest, abdomen and pelvis may be imaged in a matter of seconds, well within a single breath-hold.

Each element of the volumetric data set (voxel) in CT is, in effect, a measure of its density, and is assigned a density measurement relative to water (Hounsfield unit, after Sir Godfrey Hounsfield, an early pioneer of CT). The data set may be presented differently to assess the lung parenchyma, soft tissues, brain, bones and so on. The data produced by the CT study may be reconstructed in to any plane (coronal, sagittal, oblique or curved) or manipulated to give 3-D images.

Magnetic resonance imaging

In MRI, the patient is placed in a high-strength uniform magnetic field, usually of the order of 0.5–3.0 Tesla. As a consequence, the protons within nuclei (which are spinning, electrically charged particles) align with the magnetic field to some degree. The vast majority of clinical imaging involves the hydrogen atom, which consists

Radiology: Clinical Cases Uncovered. By A. S. Shaw, E. M. Godfrey, A. Singh and T. F. Massoud. Published 2009 by Blackwell Publishing. ISBN 978-1-4051-8474-8.

of a single proton, although many nuclides possess the property of nuclear magnetic resonance. Radiofrequency waves of a specific frequency and duration are applied to the body and the spinning protons are deflected as they absorb the radiofrequency energy. Under the influence of the magnetic field, the protons then emit radiofrequency waves as they return to the aligned position. The signal generated depends upon the molecular structures involved and the local milieu. Unlike plain films and CT, MRI is not a map of density, but rather a map of hydrogen atoms and their molecular attachments (particularly fat and water). More complex sequences of radiofrequency impulses may be used to determine other properties of the tissues, for example to suppress the signal from fat or water in order to make other structures stand out.

Before a patient, or clinician, enters the high-strength magnetic field, it is imperative that they complete a safety questionnaire. The magnetic field may cause dysfunction of pacemaker devices, and heating or movement of metallic objects within the body (e.g. shrapnel, older cerebral aneurysm clips, intra-ocular foreign bodies). Modern surgical and radiological implants are usually MRI-compatible. Before entering an MRI suite, all metallic objects and items with a magnetic strip (e.g. credit card) should be removed. Loose metallic objects in the magnetic field will be propelled at high speed in to the magnet, resulting in serious injury or even death if there is a patient inside. In the event of a medical emergency, it is usual practice for the MRI staff to remove the patient from the magnet for the medical team to assess in a safe place.

Ultrasound

Sound waves of a high frequency (>20 kHz), inaudible to humans, are referred to as ultrasound. In the setting of diagnostic radiology, sound waves of 2–15 MHz are typically utilized. In order to generate the sound waves, an alternating voltage is applied within the ultrasound probe. This causes the crystals to contract or expand to a degree proportional to the voltage applied (piezoelectric effect). Repeated expansion and contraction causes pressure (sound) waves to form and the frequency of these can be controlled. Unlike X-rays or gamma-rays, ultrasound waves may be focused by manipulation of the timing of when each crystal contracts or expands. The sound waves are transmitted in to the body where they undergo reflection and refraction as they pass through the tissues and at tissue interfaces.

The reflected sound waves are absorbed by the crystals in the probe and the pressure waves create an electrical voltage (the exact opposite of generating the sound wave). The ultrasound machine uses these signals to build up an image in real-time of very high resolution, greater than that seen in CT or MRI. Low frequency (2–5 MHz) probes are used to examine deeper structures (liver, kidneys), while superficial tissues (e.g. tendons, muscle, thyroid) are examined with higher frequency probes. The higher the frequency used, the greater the resolution, but with a consequent reduction in the depth of tissues that can be examined.

Ultrasound does not involve any ionizing radiation and, at the energies used in diagnostic imaging, has no biological effects on human tissue. Increasingly, higher energy ultrasound is being utilized in other clinical settings. Musculoskeletal injuries may occasionally be treated using ultrasound; in essence, the tissues are being heated by the deposition of energy at the site of an injury in an attempt to increase blood flow and improve tissue healing. The logical progression of this has been the development of high-intensity focused ultrasound (HIFU), where practitioners focus very high energy ultrasound on a focal site of tumour over a period of time (often hours). This effectively 'cooks' the tissue concerned and thus may help to treat or palliate patients with malignancy. Early results are promising, but it is one of a number of competing technologies in this field.

Fluoroscopy/contrast studies

This is a generic term to cover investigations where a high density material (contrast agent) is injected or introduced in to a bodily cavity and a series of radiographs then performed to outline the anatomy and, occasionally, function of a particular organ. Their use in recent years has declined significantly as clinicians and radiologists use alternative imaging methods. The barium swallow (oesophagus), meal (stomach and duodenum) and enema (colon) have largely been replaced by endoscopy. Intravenous urography has become CT urography, while the biliary system is better imaged with ultrasound and MRI techniques. Evaluation of the small bowel remains difficult. The small bowel follow through (patient swallows liquid barium) or small bowel enema (liquid barium injected via a naso-jejunal tube) are gradually being replaced in many centres by CT, MRI and capsule endoscopy.

Despite this, there remain a number of areas in which contrast studies are used. In paediatric imaging, contrast studies are frequently used to investigate the gastrointestinal system (e.g. malrotation, gastro-oesophageal reflux) and renal tract (e.g. vesico-ureteric reflux). Following surgery, contrast studies may be helpful in looking at the integrity of anastamoses.

Interventional radiology

This term covers a broad range of procedures whereby a radiologist will introduce needles, wires and/or catheters in to the vascular system, solid organs or gastrointestinal tract under imaging guidance. Such studies may be diagnostic in their own right (e.g. angiogram of the legs), be performed in order to obtain tissue for pathological analysis (i.e. ultrasound, CT or MRI-guided biopsy), or be therapeutic. This latter group has increased significantly in recent years: endovascular repair of aortic aneurysms using stent insertion in place of open surgery; coil embolization of cerebral aneurysms rather than operative clipping; and colonic stent insertion for palliation in colonic cancer to avoid surgery are just three examples of the diverse nature of this specialty. Advances in interventional radiology are having a major impact on clinical practice in many areas.

Nuclear medicine

Unlike other modalities in radiology, the source of radiation in nuclear medicine studies is administered to the patient and the radioactive emissions detected externally to produce an image. The agents used in imaging have two basic components to their structure: a molecule that will be taken up by the end organ or pathological tissue of interest, and a radioactive isotope, most commonly one that emits gamma-rays. Because molecules are used that mimic normal biological agents, nuclear medicine studies provide functional information about the tissues. For example, a patient undergoing bone scintigraphy will receive an intravenous injection of a radio-labelled molecule that will be taken up by bone. Areas with increased physiological function will take up more tracer and the scintigram will show a 'hot spot'. Such physiological changes may be detected before any abnormalities arise on other radiological studies.

More recently, positron emission tomography (PET) has become widely clinically available. This uses a glucose analogue that enters the glycolytic pathway and emits positrons (positively charged electrons) (Fig. A). These positrons interact with an electron almost immediately, are annihilated and produce two gamma-rays, each with an energy of 511 keV, that travel in opposite directions.

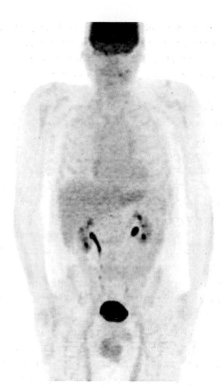

Figure A Coronal 18F-fluorodeoxyglucose positron emission tomography (FDG-PET) image demonstrating normal tracer distribution.

Radioactive emissions are detected using a bank of detectors which may be adjacent to the organ (e.g. thyroid), covering a section of the body (e.g. bone scintigram) or surrounding the body in a ring (e.g. PET). As the radiation source is not a focal point, the spatial resolution in nuclear medicine is markedly lower than that seen in other modalities, often quoted to be of the order of 5–10 mm, depending on the study. Hybrid systems, combining PET or other nuclear medicine techniques with CT allow the fusion of anatomical and physiological images. These are being increasingly utilized to guide management in a number of conditions, particularly in the field of oncology.

In addition to the diagnostic capabilities, some tumours (e.g. thyroid) may be treated by administering significantly higher doses of a radio-labelled agent. This effectively destroys the tissues in to which there is uptake.

Contrast media

Contrast media are used in radiology for a number of reasons. They may enable or enhance depiction of the

PART 1: BASICS

patient's anatomy, provide functional information about an organ system or enable the radiologist to differentiate between lesions based on their vascular characteristics.

Gastrointestinal tract studies

Plain radiographs of the chest and abdomen reveal little, if any, information regarding the gastrointestinal tract until the pathology is advanced. The use of oral or rectal contrast medium, either alone (single contrast) or in combination with air or CO_2 (double contrast), enables the radiologist to delineate the mucosal surface of the entire gastrointestinal tract. The pattern and location of any abnormalities may provide clues to the final diagnosis. The contrast agents used are barium sulphate suspension or a water-soluble iodine-based agent.

Barium studies typically give better quality images, but should be avoided if there is any suspicion of visceral perforation. The escape of barium in to the peritoneal cavity has 50% mortality, with extensive adhesions and granuloma formation in many of those who survive. Mediastinal leakage is similarly hazardous, but aspiration in to the lungs is fairly harmless and requires only physiotherapy. Water-soluble agents (e.g. gastrograffin, Gastromiro) often give inferior images because of their lower molecular weight and the effects of dilution. Older hyperosmolar agents may lead to diarrhoea and volume loss, or pulmonary oedema if aspirated. These problems are less evident with new low-osmolar agents. Water-soluble contrast medium is safe in both the mediastinum and peritoneal cavity.

Computed tomography

CT generates images with a high spatial resolution and will clearly demonstrate structures of different density (air, fat, soft tissue, calcium). This natural tissue contrast is exploited in several clinical scenarios, e.g. evaluating a pulmonary nodule (soft tissue/air) or renal calculus (calcium/soft tissue). Unfortunately, there is generally insufficient contrast when evaluating tissues of similar density, e.g. a focal lesion within the liver (soft tissue/soft tissue) or when there is a paucity of intra-abdominal fat. Consequently, patients undergoing CT are frequently given oral and/or intravenous contrast medium as part of a protocol tailored to a specific clinical question.

Oral contrast medium enables close examination of the gastrointestinal tract and may help differentiate loops of bowel from adjacent structures. Positive (high density) oral contrast agents have long been the mainstay, with most centres using a dilute solution of a water-soluble

agent (e.g. 15 mL gastrograffin/1 L water). Cordial may be added to mask the aniseed flavour of the gastrograffin. The advent of faster CT technology with greater resolution has led to the increased use of negative contrast agents. Water is the most commonly used agent, with the aim being to distend the stomach and proximal small bowel. This enables more accurate evaluation of these and adjacent structures, notably the pancreas, without obscuring subtle areas of calcification or enhancement following intravenous contrast medium. Other negative contrast agents have been described, most notably methylcellulose. This may be infused via a nasogastric tube to give distension of the small bowel (CT enteroclysis).

The intravenous contrast media used in CT are iodine-based agents which are excreted by the kidneys. As these agents pass through the pulmonary and then the systemic vasculature, the high density iodine in solution enables evaluation of the blood vessels for the presence of emboli, stenoses, aneurysms and dissection. The imaging is timed to coincide with maximum opacification of the vessels of interest. Similarly, the length of time from injection to arrival of the contrast agent in a given organ is relatively predictable. The CT is, in effect, a snapshot of the perfusion of the organs at a given time. This is crucial in imaging the abdominal viscera, where solid lesions often exhibit enhancement patterns different from the underlying organ. As a result, CT becomes a much more sensitive investigation for the detection of lesions, and in some cases the pattern of enhancement may be pathognomonic. Consequently, some CT studies may consist of multiple phases in order to determine the changes in vascularity over time. Examples of this can be seen in Fig. B.

In neuroradiology, abnormal enhancement following administration of contrast medium usually indicates disruption of the normal blood–brain barrier; the timing of imaging is not critical in this context. Recently, the use of serial imaging of the brain following administration of contrast medium has been performed. The images produced track the changes in density in the brain as the blood circulates. With this information, one is able to produce maps of cerebral perfusion to identify the early stage of an acute stroke, to assess the extent of ischaemia and thus guide therapy. This is a more accurate technique than conventional imaging alone, which may be normal or near-normal in the acute phase.

- Over the past two decades, the intravenous contrast media in common use has evolved from ionic, high osmolar solutions to non-ionic, low- or iso-osmolar

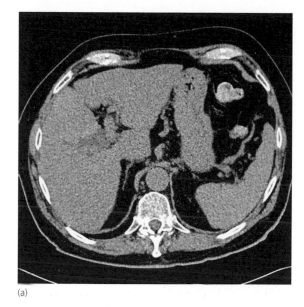

(a)

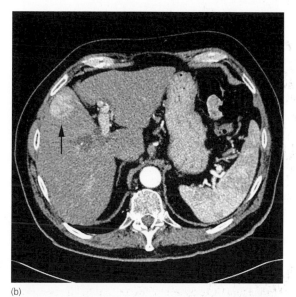

(b)

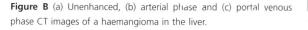

(c)

Figure B (a) Unenhanced, (b) arterial phase and (c) portal venous phase CT images of a haemangioma in the liver.

agents. This has significantly reduced the frequency of adverse clinical events associated with its use, but there remain a number of potential complications which need to be emphasized. Allergy to iodinated contrast media is not uncommon: patients may exhibit a range of symptoms from an urticarial rash to frank anaphylaxis and anaphylactoid reaction. Premedication with corticosteroids has been widely used in the past, but there is little evidence to support it and the practice has largely been discontinued. Iodinated contrast media is nephrotoxic and should be used with great care in patients with impaired renal function. The risk–benefit will need to be assessed on a case-by-case basis by the clinician and radiologist, but adequate hydration and careful monitoring of renal function is essential to minimize risk. Diabetic patients who are being treated with metformin may require temporary withdrawal of the drug following iodinated contrast media injection because of the risk of lactic acidosis; each case should be discussed with a radiologist as management will depend on the volume of

---

Box A Contraindications to CT

CT
There are no contraindications to CT *per se*, but the relative radiation risks and benefits should be emphasized in young people and pregnant women

Contrast media
- Allergy to iodine-based contrast agents
- Renal failure
- Metformin therapy may need to be temporarily halted, depending on renal function

---

Box B Contraindications to MRI

MRI
- Implanted electrical devices
- Non-compatible surgical clips/coils
- Metallic foreign bodies, e.g. shrapnel
- Pregnancy: imaging is avoided within the first trimester where possible

Contrast media
- Renal failure
- Known allergy
- Pregnancy

---

contrast medium used and the renal function of the patient. Pregnant patients and nursing mothers may be safely given intravenous contrast media, but in the case of the former, fetal thyroid activity may be suppressed and should be checked in the first week of life. Of note, the same agents are used in intravenous urography (IVU/IVP), venography and interventional radiology procedures.

Magnetic resonance imaging

There are a number of contrast agents available for use in MRI, all of which result in changes in the local magnetic field. The agents in most frequent clinical use are gadolinium-based paramagnetic (i.e. weakly magnetic) agents. They predominantly affect the protons in water molecules, shortening T1 relaxation time and producing high signal intensity on T1-weighted images. Gadolinium agents may be injected intravenously and pass through the vascular system in a similar manner to iodine-based agents. Some agents exhibit hepatocyte uptake and thus may have benefits in liver imaging. Although generally considered safe, over the past decade a new entity, nephrogenic systemic fibrosis, has been described following administration of some gadolinium agents to patients in renal failure. Consequently, caution needs to be exercised in this patient group in order to minimize the risks of developing this potentially fatal disease.

Superparamagnetic agents, containing particles of iron oxide, are also in clinical use. These agents are taken up by the reticulo-endothelial system and have applications in either liver or lymph node imaging. Unlike paramagnetic agents, these are best visualized on T2-weighted images where they reduce signal intensity. Oral contrast agents are not used frequently in MRI, but both positive and negative agents are available for use in small bowel imaging, an emerging technique.

Ultrasound

Ultrasound imaging is based upon the reflection of sound waves by tissues to produce a real-time image. Different tissues, and the interfaces between adjacent tissues, reflect sound to varying degrees. Ultrasound provides very high spatial resolution images and is thus extensively used in abdominal, vascular and 'small parts' (thyroid, testes, musculoskeletal) imaging. The past decade has seen the introduction of ultrasound contrast media in many countries, particularly across Europe. These consist of inert 'microbubbles' measuring $2–6\,\mu m$ in diameter made from a variety of biocompatible materials that contain a high molecular weight, low solubility gas, in solution. Microbubbles are stable for several minutes and are highly reflective of ultrasound. Injected intravenously, microbubbles remain within the vascular space. They have been most widely used in liver imaging in order to demonstrate vascular patency and to identify and characterize focal lesions. Numerous other applications have been described from acute abdominal trauma and inflammatory bowel disease to differentiation of benign and malignant breast tumours. Non-vascular applications described include assessment of vesico-ureteric reflux in children and fallopian tube patency in adults. Ultrasound contrast agents are generally considered safe in the majority of clinical situations. However, there have been recent reports associating their use with cardiac events in patients with pre-existing cardiac disease and thus caution should be exercised in this patient group.

Radiation exposure in diagnostic radiology

Each of us is exposed to ionizing radiation constantly, from radioactive materials in the environment and from space. The amount to which we are exposed depends upon our geographical location and altitude. Patients who undergo an X-ray, CT or nuclear medicine study will be exposed to ionizing radiation in a controlled situation. The precise dose for any given examination will depend on a number of variables including the equipment used and the technique employed. In nuclear medicine, the amount of radioactive material administered and patient metabolism will also have an effect. The typical radiation dose for each procedure is given in Table A, together with the approximate equivalent time in background radiation. This latter measure is considerably easier than effective dose for both patients and clinicians to understand when deciding upon methods of investigation.

The risk to an individual arising from exposure to ionizing radiation can be divided in to *deterministic* and *stochastic* effects. Deterministic effects are predictable consequences that will follow exposure above a certain threshold and are dose-related above that threshold. These should not be seen in diagnostic radiology but may occur in the radiotherapy setting. The effective dose of radiation delivered to the patient, from which one may predict the biological effects, is measured in sieverts (Sv), with most radiological procedures measured in millisieverts (mSv). Erythema and dry desquamation of the skin occurs at 4 Sv exposure and a similar dose to the gonads will result in sterilization. A cumulative dose of 5 Sv to the eyes results in the development of cataracts in the lens. By contrast, stochastic effects are those abnormalities that may be induced by chance, and refer almost exclusively to the induction of cancer. These probabilistic effects are thought to be dose-related, but without a threshold and thus there is no completely safe level of ionizing radiation. The risk associated with irradiation varies from organ to organ, and has been extrapolated from data generated by much higher levels of radiation exposure (particularly nuclear weapon use). Moreover, the latent period between exposure and development of cancer varies from a few years for leukaemia to decades for the solid organ tumours: many patients will die before these tumours manifest clinically. Current opinion suggests that the estimated attributable lifetime cancer mortality risk from a single whole body CT in a middle-aged patient is of the order of 1 in 1250, or 0.08%. The degree of risk will, of course, increase with repeated examinations.

There is no evidence to suggest that irradiation of an individual exposes their descendants to any genetic abnormality. The descendants of those exposed to high levels of radiation in Hiroshima and Nagasaki have not shown any difference in the frequency of congenital abnormality or in life expectancy.

Clearly, in the vast majority of cases, the potential benefit of the investigation should outweigh any potential risks. However, these risks are significantly greater in younger patients and, where possible, the exposure to ionizing radiation should be minimized or avoided altogether.

Radiology: Clinical Cases Uncovered. By A. S. Shaw, E. M. Godfrey, A. Singh and T. F. Massoud. Published 2009 by Blackwell Publishing. ISBN 978-1-4051-8474-8.

Table A The typical radiation dose for each procedure, and the approximate equivalent period of background radiation.

Procedure	Typical effective dose (mSv)	Approximate equivalent period of background radiation
Limbs/joints	<0.01	1.5 days
Chest X-ray	0.02	3 days
Skull	0.06	9 days
Hip	0.4	2 months
Abdominal X-ray	0.7	4 months
Pelvis X-ray	0.7	4 months
Lumbar spine	1.0	5 months
Barium swallow	1.5	8 months
Barium follow through	3	16 months
Barium enema	7.2	3.2 years
CT head	2.0	10 months
CT thorax	8.0	3.6 years
CT pulmonary angiogram	8.0	3.6 years
CT abdomen or pelvis	10.0	4.5 years
Lung ventilation (^{133}Xe)	0.3	7 weeks
Lung perfusion (^{99m}Tc)	1	6 months
Thyroid (^{99m}Tc)	1	6 months
Renal (^{99m}Tc)	1	6 months
Bone scintigraphy (^{99m}Tc-MDP)	4	1.8 years
Dynamic cardiac (^{99m}Tc)	6	2.7 years
FDG-PET	7	3 years
FDG-PET/CT	10–20	4.5–9 years

FDG-PET, 18F-fluorodeoxyglucose positron emission tomography.

Approach to interpreting a radiological image

Clearly, many complex radiological investigations will necessitate interpretation by a specialist. However, it is vital that physicians and surgeons from many disciplines are able to interpret basic investigations and to engage with colleagues in radiology to understand what information the other party needs and has to offer. When reviewing any radiological study, it is crucial to follow a set routine in order to minimize the risks of not identifying an abnormality. For all examinations, the following rules should be carefully observed:

1 Confirm the patient's name and date of birth on the study
2 Confirm the date and time of the study
3 Has the study been correctly imaged and labelled (left/right; supine/erect)
4 Check that you have all the current images
5 Whenever possible, compare any potentially abnormal findings with previous images. The advent of PACS (Patient Archiving and Communication Systems) in recent years has meant that previous images are now stored digitally and readily available for review

Listed below are approaches to viewing common examinations that one may encounter in clinical practice. The aim is to avoid 'blind spots' where abnormalities may be overlooked; the interpretation of abnormalities is covered in Part 2 of this book.

Skeletal X-rays

These are usually taken in patients with a history of pain, an arthropathy, following trauma or in certain systemic conditions (e.g. multiple myeloma). If there is any clinical suspicion of a fracture or dislocation, two or more views of a given bone or joint will usually be acquired in order that joint position and/or the presence of fractures may be assessed.

1 Are the bones intact?
• Fractures may be lucent, sclerotic (when impacted) or a buckling or step in the otherwise smooth cortical margin
• In children, check that ossification centres are present and correctly sited
2 Are the bones aligned normally?
• Check for evidence of subluxation or dislocation
3 Are there any erosions in or around the joint?
• Particularly in the evaluation of an arthropathy
4 Are there any focal lesions? If so, describe:
• Site
• Size
• Margins
• Matrix
• Periosteal reaction
• Soft tissue extension
5 Are the soft tissues normal?
• Check for joint effusions (especially elbow and knee)
• Soft tissue swelling may be the only sign of an occult fracture (especially cervical spine)
• Are there signs of infection (especially air pockets)?
• Are there any radio-opaque foreign bodies. Note glass and metal are radio-opaque; wood and plastic are rarely radio-opaque

There are two areas that are likely to cause confusion: the immature skeleton and the presence of normal anatomical variant. These can only be learnt through observation and experience, but where there is doubt one should cross-reference with an atlas of normal development. A copy of one of these tomes can be found in all radiology departments.

Radiology: Clinical Cases Uncovered. By A. S. Shaw, E. M. Godfrey, A. Singh and T. F. Massoud. Published 2009 by Blackwell Publishing. ISBN 978-1-4051-8474-8.

Chest X-ray

The chest radiograph is ideally taken with the patient standing facing the detector with the X-rays having passed through the patient from posterior to anterior (PA) with the X-ray tube 2 m away. The distance minimizes magnification of the cardiac outline, whereas standing enables the patient to take a good breath in and thus optimize the appearances of the lung parenchyma. If the patient has been lying down, then they should ideally be sat or stood up for several minutes before the exposure to allow redistribution of air and fluid.

Ill or infirm patients may be unable to stand for their X-ray and the image will be acquired antero-posterior (AP) with the patient sitting erect, semi-erect or even lying supine, depending on the clinical state. These factors will affect the final image and the appearances of some pathological entities. It is therefore crucial to note these factors before commenting on the remainder of the image.

1 *Lines and tubes.* Comment on the presence and position of each tube or line, e.g. where is the tip of the endotracheal or nasogastric tube? Failure to do so may have significant consequences for the patient.

2 *Cardiac size.* This can be measured in two ways on the PA film and preferences vary between clinicians. As a proportion, the heart should measure less than 50% of the thoracic diameter. Alternatively, a direct measurement of the transverse diameter can be made, with 15 cm in women and 16 cm in men considered the upper limit of normal.

3 *Mediastinal contours.* On the right, one should be able to follow (from superior to inferior) the right tracheal wall (paratracheal stripe), the great vessels (aorta, superior vena cava) and the right atrium (forming the right heart border). On the left, one can follow the tracheal wall, aortic arch, pulmonary trunk, left atrial appendage and left ventricle (the latter two forming the left heart border). The hilar vessels and main bronchi will be projected behind these on both sides as these lie in the middle mediastinum. Posteriorly, the oesophagus is not normally seen, but the lateral margin of the descending aorta should be visible.

4 *Lung parenchyma*
- Compare left with right
- Are the volumes similar?
- The pattern of a diffuse lung disease is often best assessed at the periphery of the lungs. Are there nodules, lines or rings?

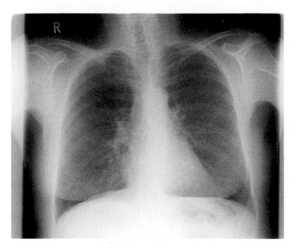

Figure C Normal PA chest radiograph.

- Are the costophrenic recesses sharp?
- Are there any pleural lesions?

5 *Bones.* Focal lesions may be difficult to identify. Turning the image through 90° so the ribs are vertical may help identify fractures.

6 *Soft tissues.* In a woman, are the breast shadows present? This may give a clue to diagnosis and account for difference in lung density. Are there any abnormalities seen below the diaphragm, e.g. free gas?

7 *Review areas.* Areas of the film where abnormalities are easily missed:
- Lung apices
- Hilar regions
- Behind the heart
- Below the diaphragms
- Soft tissues

The chest film is one of the more difficult studies to interpret well. Once an abnormality (or constellation of abnormalities) has been identified, it needs to be characterized and set in the clinical context before a rational diagnosis can be reached.

Abdominal X-ray

The plain abdominal film is acquired with the patient lying supine. It is predominantly indicated for the evaluation of bowel pathology (especially obstruction, perforation, colitides) and to detect abnormal calcification (especially renal tract). In patients in whom there is a clinical suspicion of bowel perforation, this should always be performed in conjunction with an erect chest X-ray. As with other films, a systematic approach is vital:

1 *Bowel gas pattern.* Small bowel is sited centrally, has valvulae conniventes which cross the full width of the lumen, and measures <3 cm in diameter. Large bowel is found at the periphery of the abdomen, its haustral folds may not cross the full width of the lumen and it measures <5 cm in diameter. If one can see the outside margin of the bowel wall (without there being an adjacent loop), this implies there is a pneumoperitoneum (Rigler's sign). Gas outlining the kidneys or aorta is retroperitoneal. Gas may frequently be seen within the bile ducts. This can be a normal finding following surgery or interventional procedures, but may be a sign of biliary pathology. Check the hernial orifices.

2 *Abnormal calcification:*
- Gallstones (10% of calculi are radio-opaque)
- Renal calculi (>90% of calculi are radio-opaque)
- Chronic pancreatitis
- Abdominal aorta. Is it aneurysmal?
- Lymph nodes and veins (phleboliths) are often seen and are of no significance

3 *Soft tissues.* Look for calcification or air.

4 *Bones.* The lumbar vertebrae and pelvis may be assessed

Remember that the film has been acquired with the patient supine. Unlike the chest film, air/fluid levels will not be seen.

Computed tomography

The range of imaging possible with CT cannot be covered in this text, but there are a few key principles that should be borne in mind:

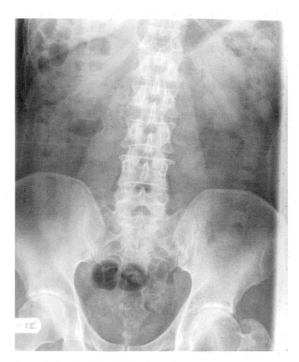

Figure D Normal abdominal radiograph.

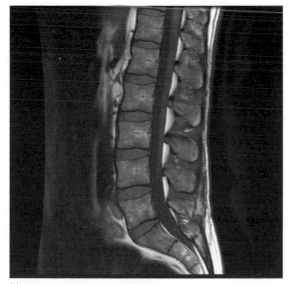 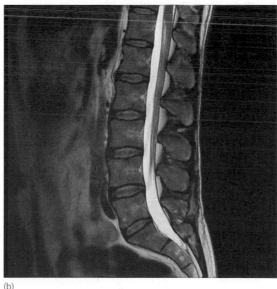

(a) (b)

Figure E Sagittal images of the lumbar spine which are (a) T1-weighted and (b) T2-weighted.

1 What part of the body has been imaged?

2 What windows have been given, e.g. bone, lung, soft tissue?

3 What plane is the imaging?

4 Has the patient been given contrast medium?
  - Oral
  - Rectal
  - Intravenous

5 What phase of contrast enhancement is it, e.g. arterial or portal venous?

With these in mind, evaluate each organ in turn, using the other side for comparison where possible, e.g. brain and thorax. Remember, the convention is for axial CT images to be presented as though one were looking up from the patient's feet, with their right on the viewer's left.

Magnetic resonance imaging

Many of the points covered in CT apply equally to MRI, although more use is made of multiplanar imaging. T1- and T2-weighted are terms related to which property of the proton spin one is examining. As a general rule, T1-weighted images give detailed anatomical information and will show fat as high signal but water as dark (e.g. cerebrospinal fluid (CSF), urine). In contrast, T2-weighted images are more sensitive for detecting pathology and will show water as high signal. The signal from any tissue may be selectively suppressed by changing the MRI sequence. Thus, key points to remember here are:

1 What sequence are you looking at, e.g. T1- or T2-weighted?

2 Have any of the tissue signals been suppressed, e.g. fat or water?

The signals from different tissues are often characteristic and it is important to look at all available sequences before coming to a conclusion.

A 58-year-old man with hemiplegia

Kevin Marshall, a 58-year-old man, presents to the accident and emergency department with a mild headache and right-sided weakness. On further questioning, Kevin had first noticed the weakness 8 hours earlier and that it had evolved rapidly such that by the time he had realized the seriousness he had been unable to reach the telephone. He was known to have mitral stenosis, but had no other past medical history. On examination, the physician found that he had a right-sided hemiplegia. Cardiovascular examination revealed a split second heart sound and quiet diastolic murmur; the pulse rate was 85 beats/minute, irregularly irregular.

What is hemiplegia?

Hemiplegia is weakness or paralysis involving the arm, leg and sometimes the face on one side of the body. It is the most common form of paralysis and is attributable to a lesion in the corticospinal pathway on the opposite side of the paralysis. The corticospinal tract starts from fibres of the motor, premotor, supplementary motor and parietal cortices, converges in the corona radiata and descends through the posterior limb of the internal capsule, cerebral peduncle, pons and medulla where 75% of the fibres decussate and the rest descend ipsilaterally as uncrossed ventral corticospinal tracts.

What are the common causes of hemiplegia?

Haemorrhagic or ischaemic vascular lesions are the most common cause of hemiplegia, followed by trauma. Other causes include tumours, demyelination, abscess and meningoencephalitis.

Radiology: Clinical Cases Uncovered. By A. S. Shaw, E. M. Godfrey, A. Singh and T. F. Massoud. Published 2009 by Blackwell Publishing. ISBN 978-1-4051-8474-8.

What is a 'stroke'?

'Stroke' is a broad term that means sudden onset of an acute neurological event attributable to a heterogeneous group of cerebrovascular disorders:
- Cerebral ischaemia and infarction (Box 1.1)
- Primary intracranial haemorrhage: intracerebral, subarachnoid, intraventricular, subdural, extradural
- Veno-occlusive disease

Why might Mr Marshall have the headache?

There are many causes of headaches, including those of vascular origin. Patients with cerebral infarction uncommonly (20%) have headache at the onset of the episode (more commonly with embolic ischaemic lesions). Occasionally, a patient with a large cerebral infarct may experience headache caused by cerebral oedema beginning as long as a few days after the onset of stroke.

Other causes of headache include: migraine, tension-type, low or high intracranial pressure, intracranial infection, trauma, drugs, metabolic disorders, systemic infections, neuralgias and pathology originating in the face and/or cranial structures.

How would you systematically appraise Mr Marshall?

It is important to use a systematic clinical approach when evaluating the patient with a potential cerebrovascular problem. In all patients in whom cerebrovascular disorders are suspected, it is useful to seek answers to four fundamental questions:

1 *Is the problem vascular?* The classic vascular setback involves a sudden onset with rapid progression to maximum neurological deficit instantaneously or in a matter of seconds. All the affected areas of the body are involved from the onset. The rapid onset and evolution usually apply to all types of cerebrovascular episodes,

> **Box 1.1 Terminology of cerebral ischaemic events**
>
> - A transient ischaemic attack (TIA) is defined as a temporary episode of focal ischaemic neurological dysfunction that completely resolves within 24 hours of onset
> - A focal ischaemic deficit that persists for longer than 24 hours but resolves within 3 weeks is a reversible ischaemic neurological deficit (RIND, considered a minor stroke)
> - If the deficit lasts longer than 3 weeks it is called cerebral infarction (an ischaemic stroke)
> - Occasionally, increasing neurological deficits may occur for as long as 72 hours after the onset of symptoms, called a progressing cerebral infarction

regardless of the total duration of symptoms, e.g. transient ischaemic attack (TIA), reversible ischaemic neurological deficit (RIND) and cerebral infarction. An exception is progressive cerebral infarction.

2 *Is the vascular problem one of haemorrhage or ischaemia?* Ischaemic strokes are more common, occurring in 80–85% of all strokes; 10% are caused by intracerebral haemorrhage and 5% by subarachnoid haemorrhage. Onset of symptoms with headache, stiff neck and diminished level of consciousness favour a haemorrhage. Ischaemia is more likely if the symptoms are of neurological dysfunction from a single arterial territory, or if improvement occurs rapidly or early in the clinical course. The distinction between them is seldom difficult clinically but sometimes the two occur simultaneously, in which case imaging may be used to distinguish the two.

3 *If the problem is haemorrhage, what is its location and cause?* Imaging can be used to distinguish the five locations of intracranial haemorrhage: intraparenchymal, intraventricular, subarachnoid, subdural and extradural.

4 *If the problem is infarction, what is the arterial or venous distribution and what is the underlying mechanism for the ischaemia?* Localizing the neurological dysfunction to one or more vascular territories requires knowledge of neuroanatomy, including that of the cerebral circulation. The first step is to distinguish generalized ischaemia (syncope, anoxic encephalopathy) from focal cerebral ischaemia (TIA, RIND, infarction, progressive infarction). If it is focal, then distinguish anterior circulation from posterior circulation insults. Next, subdivide the

lesion in to individual or multiple vascular territories. Finally, consider the underlying mechanism, whether it is caused by: (a) cardiac disease, (b) large vessel (craniocervical occlusive) disease, (c) small vessel (intracranial occlusive) disease or (d) haematological diseases. Another common way to categorize ischaemic stroke is as thrombotic infarction (where locally decreased blood supply is caused by blockage formed in an artery *in situ*), or as embolic infarction (where blockage is caused by a fragment of material that has broken free from a more proximal site).

How might Mr Marshall's history of mitral stenosis relate to his stroke?

Mitral valve disease is associated with atrial fibrillation, as was seen in this case. Atrial fibrillation is the heart arrhythmia most frequently associated with embolic brain infarction. The atria do not contract fully, resulting in stagnation of blood and predisposition to intraluminal thrombi. The risk of brain embolization increases with longer duration of the arrhythmia, especially when associated with valvular heart disease, e.g. mitral stenosis.

How would you manage this patient on presentation?

Patients with an acute stroke should be treated with the same sense of urgency as patients with an acute myocardial infarction. An ischaemic stroke is a 'brain attack' indicating an abrupt lack of blood supply to a region of the brain. Most patients presenting with cerebral infarction should be admitted to hospital for urgent evaluation and treatment.

Obtaining a detailed history is the most important part of evaluating a patient with a stroke. Approximately 80% of stroke diagnosis can be based on this. It is important to identify and characterize the following signs and symptoms:

1 The patient's main symptoms
2 Time of onset and precipitating events
3 Temporal evolution of onset of symptoms
4 Neurological deficits, whether focal or generalized, as well as any change in level of consciousness
5 Any headaches, vomiting, seizures, and
6 Temporal course or evolution (if any) of the neurological symptoms

Early after the onset of a severe deficit, it is not possible to classify the deficit as a TIA, RIND, an ischaemic stroke or a progressive stroke because it is unknown if and when the deficit might clear. However, the history and clinical examination may verify that the probable cause is an ischaemic stroke.

What radiological investigations would you request for this patient?

CT has revolutionized the clinician's ability to distinguish between haemorrhage and infarction in emergency situations. Ischaemic lesions appear as normal areas or as areas of decreased attenuation within the first several hours after the onset of symptoms, whereas haemorrhagic lesions usually appear immediately as areas of increased attenuation. CT without contrast medium is the usual initial imaging investigation because of its accessibility and rapidity. However, on admission, the CT is negative in about one-third of patients in whom an ischaemic stroke has been diagnosed clinically, e.g. the infarct may be too small or difficult to see because of proximity to skull base. Moreover, even within the first 24 hours after a stroke, the CT may be negative in about 50% of cases because of little associated oedema.

What does this initial imaging show?

There is a hyperdense left middle cerebral artery (MCA; Fig. 1.1, arrow) and relatively normal brain parenchyma (Fig. 1.2). The hyperdense MCA sign is an indirect sign of cerebral ischaemia that corresponds to occlusion of the MCA. It most likely represents occlusion of the artery by an intraluminal clot from a thrombus or embolus, and theoretically can be seen on CT images within the first 6 hours of a stroke before the changes of acute stroke are seen in the brain parenchyma. A false positive sign may be present with a high haematocrit or calcification of the artery (e.g. in diabetes). A summary of the imaging findings in cerebral infarction is given in Box 1.2.

What other techniques are available to image cerebral infarction?
Contrast enhanced CT

The blood–brain barrier is disrupted in cerebral infarcts; therefore contrast medium can leak in to them and produce enhancement. This may allow visualization of a small percentage of otherwise isodense and undetectable infarcts, especially in the second to fourth week after a stroke. After 1 month, an infarct typically will not enhance.

CT perfusion studies

This technique provides a quantitative measurement of regional cerebral blood flow by analysis of blood flow in each pixel of brain parenchyma. A perfusion CT study involves sequential acquisition of stationary brain CT sections during intravenous administration of contrast medium. Analysis of the resultant contrast enhancement curves allows the calculation of three parameters that

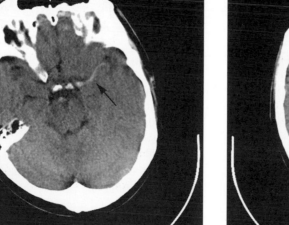
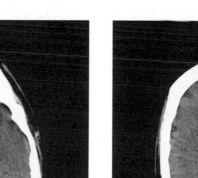

Figure 1.1 Unenhanced axial CT of the head.

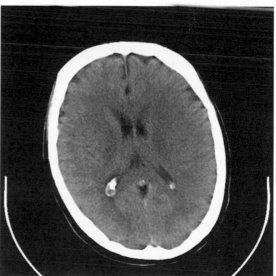

Figure 1.2 Unenhanced axial CT of the head.

Box 1.2 Imaging signs of cerebral infarction

- *In the hyperacute phase* (<6 hours): CT may be normal or there may be subtle decreased attenuation of subcortical white matter. There may be a hyperdense artery indicating its thrombosis in 25% of cases. On MRI this may be seen as absence of 'flow void' in this artery. On diffusion-weighted MRI there may be restricted diffusion (which lasts on average for the next 12 days)
- *In the acute phase* (6–24 hours): on CT there may be low density of the basal ganglia, some loss of the grey–white matter interface and early mass effect owing to the build-up of oedema. On MRI, early swelling of the cortical gyri may be seen
- *In the late acute phase* (1–3 days): on both CT and MRI, wedge-shaped infarct affecting both grey and white matter, mass effect may be seen and haemorrhagic transformation may begin
- *In the early subacute phase* (4–7 days): oedema and mass effect persist. Gyral and parenchymal enhancement may occur. Haemorrhagic transformation may become apparent
- *In the late subacute phase* (1–8 weeks): the mass effect and oedema resolves, sometimes leading to the radiological disappearance of the infarcted area. This 'fogging effect' corresponds to a period of invasion by macrophages and capillary proliferation. Enhancement may persist
- *In the chronic phase* (months to years): volume loss, atrophy and encephalomalacia, and no enhancement

---

Box 1.3 Diffusion-weighted imaging

- An MRI technique that looks at the diffusion of water in biological tissues
- This essentially images Brownian motion
- Areas of infarction show oedematous cells with restricted diffusion
- Consequently, ischaemia shows as dark areas on apparent diffusion coefficient (ADC) maps and as bright (hyperintense) areas on diffusion-weighted images

---

describe the cerebral haemodynamics in each pixel of the cerebral CT section:

1 The regional cerebral blood volume (rCBV)
2 The blood mean transit time (MTT) through cerebral capillaries, and
3 The regional cerebral blood flow (rCBF), producing semi-quantitative maps.

Perfusion CT studies are easy and quick to perform. In the future, perfusion CT studies will perhaps modify the management of acute stroke patients, for instance with respect to inclusion criteria in thrombolysis protocols.

Magnetic resonance imaging

MRI produces images that generally are more detailed (much higher spatial resolution) than those of CT and that provide more information about tissue characteristics. In many stroke cases, however, MRI does not yield information over and above CT that would alter management, but it does have some specific advantages: it is more sensitive to tissue changes (small infarcts may be detected earlier and more precisely), and there are no bony artefacts to obscure infarcts near the skull base. Indeed, MRI is considered a better test than CT for identifying acute ischaemic changes, with a specific technique (diffusion-weighted MRI; Box 1.3) being a highly specific test for early detection of usually irreversible parenchymal injury. A disadvantage of MRI relative to CT is that the study may be normal for 24 hours after intracranial haemorrhage, yet another reason for favouring the use of CT as the initial imaging technique for the acute stroke patient.

Magnetic resonance angiography

Magnetic resonance angiography (MRA) is a subtype of MRI that can non-invasively visualize extracranial and intracranial arterial and venous vessels with or without the administration of contrast medium.

What other laboratory investigations would you request for this patient?

- *Chest X-ray.* Reveals heart size and any unsuspected lung pathology.
- *Biochemical analysis.* Blood urea nitrogen, electrolytes, creatinine, cholesterol, blood glucose.
- *Haematological analysis.* Full blood count, platelets, haemoglobin, haematocrit, prothrombin time, partial thromboplastin time and other tests that may be used for specific haematological disorders.
- *Cardiac assessment.* The heart and carotid arteries should be examined clinically in all patients with cerebrovascular disease. Electrocardiography may reveal

evidence of myocardial ischaemia or infarction, arrhythmias or left ventricular hypertrophy as a potential cause of ischaemic stroke or TIA. Echocardiography may be needed to quickly evaluate cardiac anatomy.
• *Colour-coded duplex ultrasound study of neck arteries.* A useful technique for rapid identification of patients at high risk from stenosis of the carotid bifurcation.

What are the next steps in clinical management?

Subsequent management includes:

1 Intensive general medical care
2 Treatment of neurological deficits
3 Prevention of subsequent neurological events
4 Prevention and treatment of secondary complications such as pneumonia, urinary tract infection and deep vein thrombosis

If the history and examination verified that the probable cause of the hemiplegia in this patient was an ischaemic stroke, and if the onset of symptoms had been less than 3–6 hours before the evaluation, emergency thrombolytic therapy (e.g. using tissue plasminogen activator) should have been considered. However, the late presentation of the patient precluded this, and therefore the initial therapeutic approach included consideration of the use of heparin. Patients with small or moderate infarcts may be safely anticoagulated if the activated partial thromboplastin time is monitored closely. With large infarcts involving the entire MCA or internal carotid artery distribution, heparin is usually withheld early and repeated imaging is obtained several days after the onset of symptoms. If there is no evidence of haemorrhagic transformation, treatment may involve intravenous heparin and close monitoring of the activated partial thromboplastin, or warfarin. Other emergency treatments of acute stroke include several categories of neuroprotective agents designed to limit or reverse parenchymal damage.

If atrial fibrillation is a new finding at the time the patient presents with an ischaemic cerebral event, conversion to normal sinus rhythm may be indicated. Anticoagulant therapy should precede conversion because conversion itself is associated with a risk of embolization.

Mr Marshall was admitted to hospital and supportive care instituted. Seven hours after his admission, further CT imaging was performed.

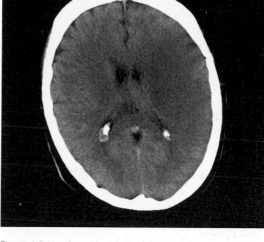

Figure 1.3 Unenhanced axial CT of the head.

What does the repeated follow-up imaging show?

The repeat CT scan 7 hours after admission shows development of extensive low density in the territory normally supplied by the left MCA, indicating early subacute infarction (Fig. 1.3). Early mass effect caused by parenchymal swelling is evident.

At this time a CT perfusion study was performed, showing a large area of unrecordable time to peak flow, and marked reduction in cerebral blood volume and flow in the left frontal and temporal lobes, as well as the insula and basal ganglia, corresponding to the area of infarction (Plates 1–3).

Mr Marshall made slow progress on the ward. One week later, an MRI study of the brain was performed.

What do these images show?

The axial FLAIR image (Fig. 1.4) confirmed the presence of a large established left MCA territory infarct, which corresponds to restricted diffusion on the diffusion-weighted imaging (Fig. 1.5). An MRA at this time showed recanalization of the left MCA (Fig. 1.6, arrow).

The hyperdense MCA sign is a transient phenomenon, as suggested in serial CT studies. In most patients this sign is absent 1 week later, which confirms the mobile nature of the clot.

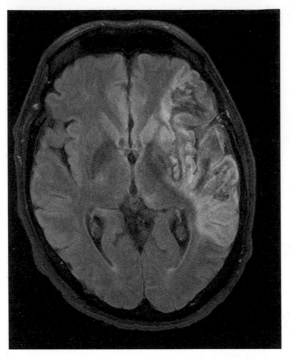

Figure 1.4 Axial T2-weighted FLAIR image. This sequence is T2-weighted but suppresses cerebrospinal fluid (CSF) signal.

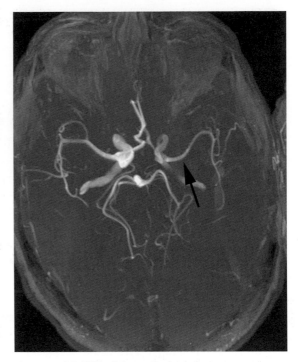

Figure 1.6 3-D MRA of the cerebral vessels.

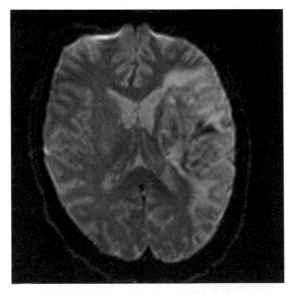

Figure 1.5 Axial diffusion-weighted image of the brain.

What is the prognosis for Mr Marshall?

Survival after the first cerebral infarction is about 65% at 1 year, 50% at 5 years, 30% at 8 years and 25% at 10 years. The most common causes of death after a cerebral infarct are transtentorial herniation, pneumonia, cardiac disorders, pulmonary embolus and septicaemia. Death occurs most commonly on day 1 or 2 after the onset of an infarct, and considerably less frequently after day 7.

Motor recovery tends to occur in the first 2–3 months, and leg improvement is usually better than arm movement. In patients with hemiparesis, about 20% have persistent severe hemiparesis at 6 months after the event, whereas 50% have a perceptible weakness at 1 year.

CASE REVIEW

Kevin Marshall is a 58-year-old man who presented to the accident and emergency department with an 8-hour history of headache and rapidly progressive right-sided weakness. He was known to have mitral stenosis and on clinical examination it was discovered that he now had atrial fibrillation. He had a right-sided hemiplegia. He was immediately referred for a CT of the head which identified a hyperdense thrombus within the left MCA although the brain parenchyma looked normal.

Supportive care was instituted and several hours later the imaging was repeated with a perfusion study also performed. By this stage, a large left MCA territory infarct was evident and the perfusion study shows the classic features of infarction.

Mr Marshall made slow progress over the course of the next week, at which stage an MRI study was able to demonstrate recanalization of the MCA, but on the background of an established MCA territory infarction.

KEY POINTS

- Acute cerebral ischaemic events may be reversible if they present early
- Clinical history should establish the time of onset and symptoms
- Urgent imaging should be performed to ascertain the cause of focal neurological deficits
- The signs of infarction at CT vary according to the age of the infarction
- Perfusion imaging may help identify areas of infarction and reversible ischaemia not apparent on conventional CT images
- MRI is not commonly used in the acute setting, but may be used as a problem-solving tool
- Investigations should be directed towards identifying an underlying cause where possible
- Thrombolysis may be used to treat ischaemia in certain circumstances
- Clinical management is otherwise supportive in the first instance

Case 2 | A 65-year-old woman with visual disturbance, headaches and vomiting

Janet Miller, a 65-year-old woman with a past history of breast cancer, presents to her local hospital accident and emergency department with several weeks of persistent headaches and some deterioration in her vision which she had thought were caused by migraine. She had started vomiting 3 days before presentation. Examination of Mrs Miller's eyes confirmed that she had decreased visual acuity at 6/20. Further, her visual fields were markedly abnormal with a left homonymous hemianopia. Following the clinical examination, the doctor concluded that there were signs of raised intracranial pressure (ICP).

What are the clinical signs of raised intracranial pressure?

The initial signs of raised ICP are non-specific and include headache and vomiting. However, as this progresses the clinical signs become more pronounced. These are given in Box 2.1.

Why does raised intracranial pressure occur?

The intracranial cavity is a non-compliant space of fixed volume. It contains brain, blood, cerebrospinal fluid (CSF) and supporting dura. The intracranial space is separated in to compartments by rigid dural layers. Because the compliance of both the total space and the subcompartments is limited, pressures can increase rapidly as a result of small changes in volumes of contents, and herniation between compartments or through the foramen magnum may ensue. Conversely, dramatic decreases in pressure can result from small decreases in contents, which is the principal underlying medical management of raised ICP. The various potential causes of raised ICP are given in Box 2.2.

Radiology: Clinical Cases Uncovered. By A. S. Shaw, E. M. Godfrey, A. Singh and T. F. Massoud. Published 2009 by Blackwell Publishing. ISBN 978-1-4051-8474-8.

Mrs Miller is referred urgently for a CT of the head.

What does this image show?

There is a large mass (Fig. 2.1, arrow) arising posteriorly and within the right occipital lobe which is distorting the brain parenchyma.

What are the causes of intracranial masses?

1 *Malignancy.* Metastases, gliomas, meningiomas, pituitary adenomas and acoustic neuromas account for 95% of all brain tumours. In adults, two-thirds of primary brain tumours are supratentorial, but in children, two-thirds of brain tumours are infratentorial. Primary tumours include astrocytomas, glioblastoma multiforme, oligodendrogliomas and ependymomas. About 30% of brain tumours are metastatic deposits and of these about 50% are multiple. About 15–20% of patients with metastatic cancer develop cerebral metastases. The most common primary is lung cancer followed by breast cancer, carcinoma of the colon and malignant melanoma.

2 *Other space occupying lesions.* A haematoma may follow trauma. Risk factors include old age and anticoagulation. Cerebral abscesses are uncommon but risk factors include chronic obstructive pulmonary disease (COPD), which may be a source of infection to the systemic circulation, and a right to left shunt that permits infection to bypass the lungs which would normally filter it out. Cerebral abscesses are multiple in 25% of cases. Cerebral amoebiasis and cysticercosis are rare. Both infection and lymphomas of the CNS are more common with HIV infection. Granulomas and tuberculomas can occur.

3 Focal CNS pathology that may have mass effect:
- Stroke
- Traumatic contusion
- Vasculitis
- Multiple sclerosis
- Encephalitis

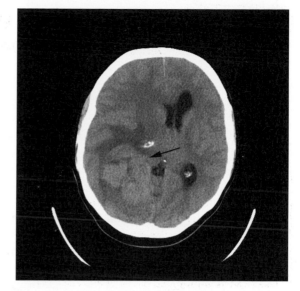

Figure 2.1 Unenhanced axial CT of the head.

Why does Mrs Miller have a hemianopia?

A lesion of the optic tract behind the chiasm disconnects fibres from half of each retina. If the right optic tract is destroyed, visual function is lost in the right halves of both retinae. However, the result is described with reference to the defect that is produced in the visual fields. In this instance there is blindness for objects in the left half of each field of vision, i.e. a left homonymous hemianopia. Lesions that destroy the entire visual area of the right occipital lobe, or all the fibres of the right optic radiation, will also produce a left homonymous hemianopia.

How would you manage her raised intracranial pressure?

Management is directed towards the underlying disease:
- Excision of primary tumours, with additional radiotherapy and chemotherapy if necessary

- Palliative care is usually required for metastases. This may include radiotherapy. However, surgery may be contemplated with up to three metastases
- Haematoma may need evacuation
- Infectious lesions will usually need both evacuation and antibiotic therapy
- Other treatments may be required either as part of radical treatment, as palliative care, or both:
  - elevate head of bed
  - dexamethasone can reduce cerebral oedema
  - mannitol may reduce raised intracranial pressure
  - anticonvulsants may be required but should not be given prophylactically before fits occur
  - treat headache with codeine phosphate as it avoids the pupillary effect of opiates
  - avoid hypotension in order to maintain cerebral perfusion pressure
  - may need to intubate and hyperventilate

What further radiological investigations would you request for Mrs Miller?

MRI is the modality of choice in the evaluation of primary brain tumours and metastases, as it allows more accurate delineation of tumour margins and provides more information with which to differentiate between various tumour types. Overall, when compared with CT, MRI has a much greater range of available soft tissue contrast, depicts anatomy in greater detail and is more

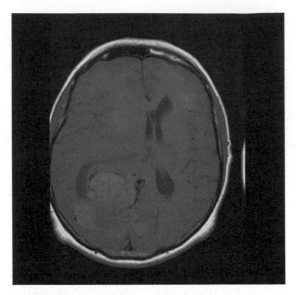

Figure 2.2 Axial T1-weighted image through the brain.

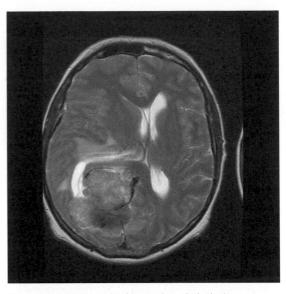

Figure 2.4 Axial T2-weighted image through the brain.

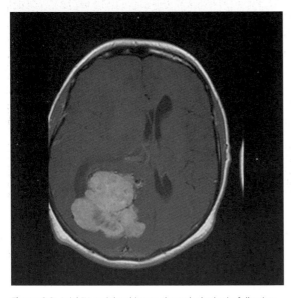

Figure 2.3 Axial T1-weighted image through the brain following intravenous gadolinium.

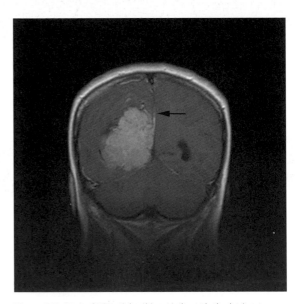

Figure 2.5 Coronal T1-weighted image through the brain following intravenous gadolinium.

sensitive and specific for abnormalities within the brain itself.

What does this MRI scan show?

There is a large (6 cm maximum diameter, Figs 2.2–2.5) lobulated mass postero-medial to the trigone of the right lateral ventricle, in the region of the right occipital lobe. This mass is of heterogeneous signal intensity on T1 and

T2-weighted images, showing strong but heterogeneous enhancement after contrast administration. A dural tail is seen along the posterior falx (Fig. 2.5, arrow). The mass crosses the midline and is surrounded by extensive oedema, resulting in marked mass effect on the nearby right lateral ventricle, and a 1 cm right to left midline shift.

In interpreting the imaging findings of an intracranial mass it is important first to decide if a lesion is intra-axial (intraparenchymal) or extra-axial (outside the brain tissue, i.e. meningeal, dural, epidural or intraventricular). The implications in terms of pathology and treatment of the mass are different depending on this location. The most common extra-axial mass is meningioma, which is also intradural. It therefore buckles white matter, expands adjacent subarachnoid space and may cause bony reactive changes. Seeing the dural margin often determines that the lesion is extra-axial. A typical extra-axial but extradural mass is a bone metastasis, which may displace the dura inward. Intra-axial lesions expand the brain cortex and dura is peripheral to the mass. It may be difficult to distinguish intra-axial from extra-axial lesions when masses are very large or aggressively invade their surroundings.

What is the differential diagnosis?

Malignancy is the most likely on account of the aggressive appearances of the mass. It incites extensive oedema and results in marked mass effect, it is lobulated and with irregular margins and it enhances heterogeneously. Breast cancer metastasis or a glioma would be most likely. The tumour also abuts the dura of the posterior falx cerebri, which therefore also raises the possibility of an extra-axial aggressive tumour such as a metastasis or a malignant meningioma.

What is the next step in clinical management?

Surgical excision to relieve raised ICP, and also to obtain tissue diagnosis.

Mrs Miller underwent a craniotomy and resection of the lesion. Histology of the lesion showed it to be an anaplastic meningioma (Box 2.3). Owing to the aggressive nature of the tumour Mrs Miller subsequently underwent a course of radiotherapy.

Is this the usual presentation of this disease?

No. More than 90% of meningiomas are benign tumours. They therefore grow very slowly, often over many years; they can sometimes become extremely large before being detected (Figs 2.6–2.8). Meningiomas are often diagnosed on a CT or MRI scan based on a patient's symptoms, e.g. seizures, focal weakness, sensory loss or cranial nerve (including visual) deficit. However, many meningiomas are discovered as 'incidental' findings when a patient is scanned for an unrelated complaint, e.g. after

> **Box 2.3 Malignant meningioma**
>
> - Meningiomas are tumours that arise from the leptomeninges, i.e. are of meningothelial origin, from arachnoid cap cells
> - Typical benign meningiomas are found in >90% of cases
> - Atypical meningioma (having intermediate hypercellularity and mitotic activity) and anaplastic meningioma (malignant, with brain invasion) occur in <10%
> - The diagnosis is usually made postoperatively
> - Treatment is a combination of surgery and radiotherapy
> - There is no role for chemotherapy

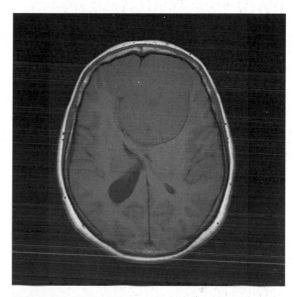

Figure 2.6 Axial T1-weighted image of the brain.

a CT scan has been performed in the setting of head trauma.

Meningiomas are the second most common primary brain tumour after astrocytomas, and are the most common intracranial extra-axial tumours. They occur more often in females 40–70 years of age, and there is an association with breast cancer. They may be found in diverse locations: parasagittal, convexity, sphenoid ridge, olfactory groove, parasellar and also intraspinal. They can be multiple in 10% of cases (Figs 2.9–2.12); 3% of the population >60 years of age have an incidental meningioma at autopsy.

The imaging features of a typical meningioma are that of a mass that is discrete, rounded and hyperdense on

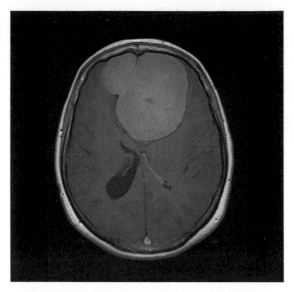

Figure 2.7 Axial T1-weighted image of the brain following intravenous gadolinium.

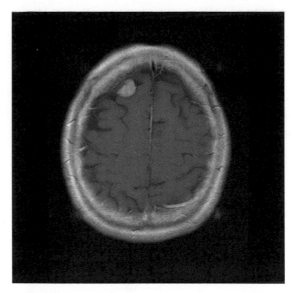

Figure 2.9 Axial T1-weighted image of the brain following intravenous gadolinium.

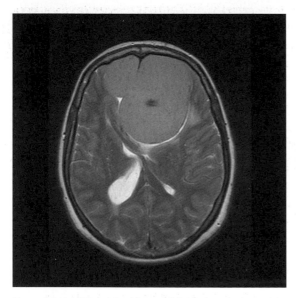

Figure 2.8 Axial T2-weighted image of the brain.

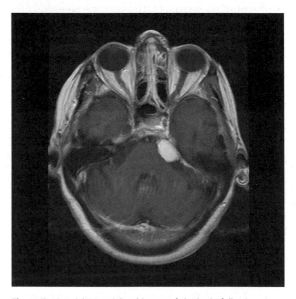

Figure 2.10 Axial T1-weighted image of the brain following intravenous gadolinium.

CT or iso-intense on MRI. It may result in adjacent hyperostosis and oedema in surrounding brain is common (in 60%) but variable. These tumours enhance strongly and homogeneously, although areas of cystic necrosis or fatty change may be present, and may contain gross calcification. Menigiomas typically abut the dural surface and a 'dural tail' may be present:

enhancement of the dura trailing off away from the mass in a crescentic fashion, and although found also in many other lesions, is associated typically with meningiomas (in 72% of cases). *En plaque* (spreading flat along the dura) or intra-osseous meningiomas that extend in to adjacent bone may be difficult to see on non-contrast imaging.

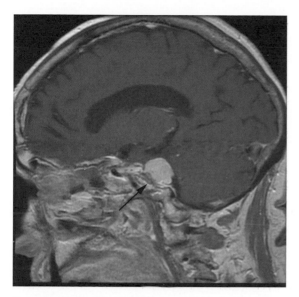

Figure 2.11 Sagittal T1-weighted image of the brain following intravenous gadolinium (meningioma arrowed).

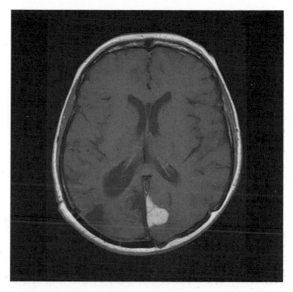

Figure 2.13 Axial T1-weighted image of the brain following intravenous gadolinium.

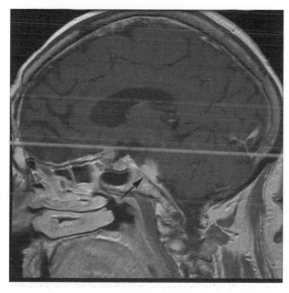

Figure 2.12 Sagittal T1-weighted image of the brain following intravenous gadolinium (arrowed).

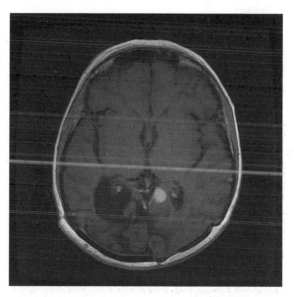

Figure 2.14 Axial T1-weighted image of the brain following intravenous gadolinium.

Meningiomas are one of the few tumours where angiography still may have a role. They are supplied by arteries arising from the dura and the pia, resulting in a delayed tumour stain (blush). Preoperative embolization may be useful to decrease the vascularity of the tumour before surgical resection.

Over the course of the next 6 years Mrs Miller was imaged at regular intervals after repeated surgery and radiotherapy. Despite this, and in keeping with the malignant nature of this meningioma, the tumour continued to spread, now on the left side of the posterior falx (Figs 2.13–2.15). She then developed a lesion at the vertex of the calvarium, which was also evaluated using MRI.

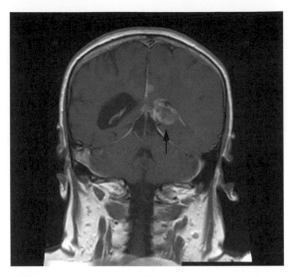

Figure 2.15 Coronal T1-weighted image of the brain following intravenous gadolinium (meningioma arrowed).

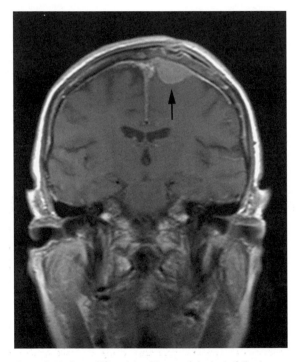

Figure 2.16 Coronal T1-weighted image of the brain following intravenous gadolinium (meningioma arrowed).

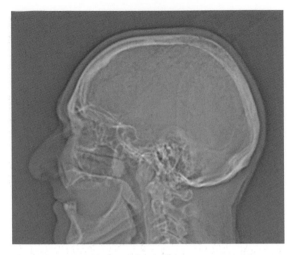

Figure 2.17 CT topogram of the skull.

What does the MRI scan of this new lesion show?

There is a large enhancing extra-axial mass in a left para-sagittal location, also abutting and spreading along the falx cerebri. It invades and expands the adjacent bone of the calvarium (Fig. 2.16).

How might you better evaluate the skull?

While MRI is of value in evaluating bone marrow, CT gives better definition of the bony cortex and periosteum.

What does this show?

The CT shows permeative destruction of the inner and outer table of the skull (arrows) by the aggressive extra-axial mass spreading in to and expanding bone (Figs 2.17 & 2.18).

What is the differential diagnosis of this new lesion?

• Intra-osseous meningioma
• Metastasis, e.g. from the previous breast cancer
• Less likely: fibrous dysplasia, myeloma, primary bone tumour

What further imaging is necessary in this patient?

A bone scan: to determine if this skull vertex lesion is solitary, which would favour the presence of a locally aggressive meningioma, as is the case here (Fig. 2.19) in

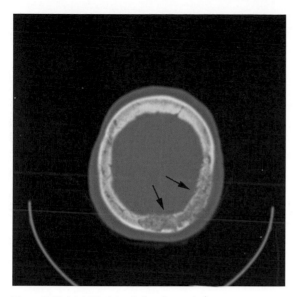

Figure 2.18 Axial CT of the skull on bony windows.

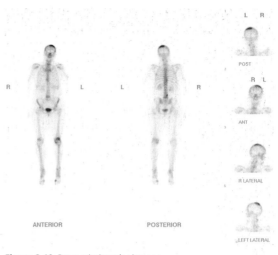

Figure 2.19 Bone scintigraphy images.

keeping with the patient's known disease, or one of many similar lesions spread throughout the body, favouring metastatic disease from her breast cancer.

Mrs Miller underwent a surgical biopsy which confirmed the lesion to be a further malignant meningioma. Mrs Miller underwent radiotherapy as the lesion was thought to be unresectable.

What is the prognosis for this disease?

This depends on location and resectability of the tumour. Overall, the 5-year recurrence is 5% for typical benign lesions, 30% for atypical and 75% for anaplastic meningiomas.

CASE REVIEW

Janet Miller, a 65-year-old woman with a past history of breast cancer presented to the accident and emergency department at her local hospital with a history of persistent headaches and gradual deterioration in her vision. She had started vomiting 3 days earlier. Examination of Mrs Miller's eyes confirmed that she had a decreased visual acuity at 6/20. Further, her visual fields were markedly abnormal with a left homonymous hemianopia. The examining clinician thought that she had signs of raised intracranial pressure and referred her immediately for a CT of the head and, subsequently, an MRI.

These images demonstrated a 6-cm lobulated mass postero-medial to the trigone of the right lateral ventricle, in the region of the right occipital lobe. A number of potential causes for the mass were determined and this was resected surgically to both relieve the raised intracranial pressure and to obtain a histological diagnosis. The lesion proved to be an anaplastic meningioma and over the next 6 years Mrs Miller underwent repeated surgical excision and radiotherapy to treat local recurrence of the disease.

Mrs Miller then developed a further lesion in a parasagittal location, spreading along the falx cerebri spreading in to and expanding bone. This was confirmed to be a solitary lesion on bone scintigraphy; surgical biopsy was undertaken and it was reported to be a second malignant meningioma. The location and extent of the lesion meant that this was not resectable and Mrs Miller was treated with further radiotherapy.

KEY POINTS

- Raised intracranial pressure may present with non-specific symptoms of headache and vomiting
- Systemic effects on the heart rate, breathing and blood pressure may ensue
- Visual examination, including fundoscopy, is essential
- It is important to have a high level of suspicion for raised ICP
- Raised ICP is a medical emergency requiring urgent imaging and treatment
- Treatment is directed towards removing the underlying cause

- Meningiomas are usually benign extra-axial lesions
- Fewer than 10% have more aggressive features on histology
- Preoperative diagnosis of atypia is rarely possible
- Treatment depends on the location and extent of the meningioma, as well as symptoms and the patient's clinical condition
- Surgical excision or radiotherapy may be used for malignant meningiomas
- Recurrence is more likely with atypical and anaplastic meningiomas

A 26-year-old woman with numb hands and feet

Susan Johnstone, a 26-year-old civil servant, presented to her general practitioner with a 1 month history of bilateral numbness in hands and feet, as well as fatigue and mild generalized motor weakness. She had noticed some blurred vision over the previous 2 weeks. She was referred for a specialist neurological opinion. On further questioning she admitted to experiencing similar but milder symptoms during the warm weather of the previous summer months.

What disease do these clinical features suggest?

Multiple sclerosis (MS) is an autoimmune disease that affects the central nervous system (CNS; the brain and spinal cord). The exact cause is not known, but MS is believed to result from damage to the myelin sheath. It is thus a primary demyelinating disease, i.e. a disorder where normal myelin is injured or destroyed but there is no accepted aetiology. The average age of onset is 30 years, but it is a progressive disease and the resulting neurodegeneration gets worse over time. In addition to nerve damage, the associated inflammation destroys the myelin, leaving multiple areas of scar tissue (sclerosis, plaques devoid of myelin). It also causes nerve impulses to slow down or stop, leading to the symptoms of MS. Repeated episodes of inflammation can occur along any area of the brain and spinal cord.

Common early symptoms include tingling, numbness, loss of balance, weakness in one or more limbs and blurred or double vision (optic neuritis). Less common symptoms may include slurred speech, sudden onset of paralysis, lack of coordination and cognitive difficulties. A history of at least two attacks separated by a period of reduced or no symptoms may be a sign of relapsing remitting MS.

Symptoms of MS may mimic many other neurological disorders. Diagnosis is made by ruling out other conditions.

What specific investigations would you request?

1 In addition to a careful neurological examination, an eye examination may show abnormal pupillary responses, changes in the visual fields or eye movements, decreased visual acuity, or problems with the internal structures of the eye. Visual (as well as auditory and somatosensory) evoked potentials are electrical diagnostic studies that measure the speed of nerve transmissions in various parts of the brain. They are sensitive to MS damage and can detect evidence of scarring along nerve pathways.

2 A lumbar puncture to obtain cerebrospinal fluid (CSF):

- *CSF oligoclonal bands.* An oligoclonal band in CSF represents a homogeneous protein secreted by a single clone of plasma cells. A single oligoclonal band is commonly seen as a normal finding. Two or more bands are considered abnormal, suggesting the presence of an immune-mediated process in the CNS. They are seen in about 90% of patients with definite MS.

- *CSF IgG index.* Increased levels of CSF immunoglobulin G (IgG) can occur with excessive production of IgG within the CNS or it can be caused by leakage of plasma proteins in to the CSF (e.g. in inflammation or trauma). To discriminate between these two possibilities, the IgG index is calculated from IgG and albumin measurements performed in CSF and serum. An elevated IgG index is found in 70–90% of MS cases.

- *Myelin basic protein* (MBP) is a product of oligodendroglia. When there is damage in the CNS, MBP can appear in the CSF (as well as blood and urine). When it is elevated in CSF it may be an additional indicator of MS.

3 Brain and spinal cord imaging. MRI is the best single method for imaging MS. It is much more sensitive than

Radiology: Clinical Cases Uncovered. By A. S. Shaw, E. M. Godfrey, A. Singh and T. F. Massoud. Published 2009 by Blackwell Publishing. ISBN 978-1-4051-8474-8.

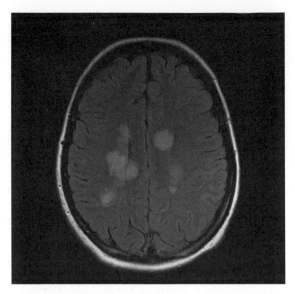

Figure 3.1 Axial FLAIR image of the brain.

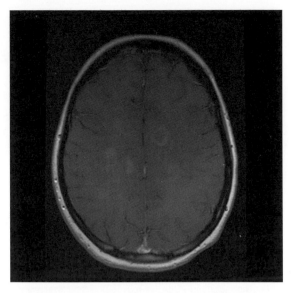

Figure 3.3 Axial T1-weighted image of the brain following intravenous gadolinium.

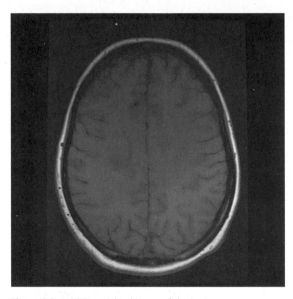

Figure 3.2 Axial T1-weighted image of the brain.

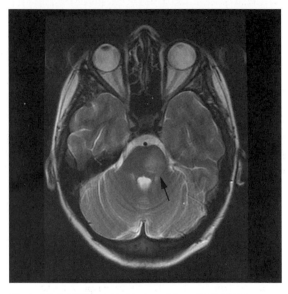

Figure 3.4 Axial T2-weighted image of the posterior fossa.

CT in detecting plaques, and can also detect spinal cord lesions (2–20% of patients with MS have cervical cord lesions and normal brain findings).

What do the MRI images show?

Figures 3.1–3.3 show multiple discrete rounded and ovoid T2 hyperintense and T1 hypointense lesions in periventricular white matter, with no significant mass effect. These lesions show variable enhancement, includ-

ing ring enhancement patterns. A large lesion is present in the left side of the pons (Fig. 3.4, arrow). Multiple areas of T2 hyperintensity are found in the mid-cervical cord (Figs 3.5 & 3.6, arrow), also resulting in cord expansion.

Are these images diagnostic of MS?

The diagnosis of MS is mainly a clinical one. The major role of imaging is:

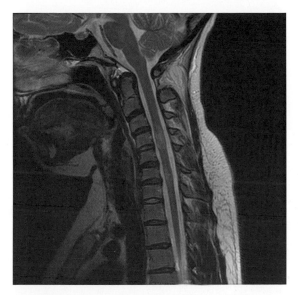

Figure 3.5 Sagittal T2-weighted image of the cervical spine.

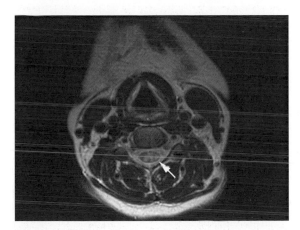

Figure 3.6 Axial T2-weighted image of the cervical spine.

1 To confirm or refute the clinical suspicion, and
2 To suggest plausible alternative diagnoses for the patient's clinical findings.

MRI alone cannot establish the diagnosis of MS. It can suggest the disease, but without supportive clinical findings other diagnoses may be more likely. These findings are, however, typical for a patient with MS (Box 3.1).

McDonald criteria

The McDonald criteria are diagnostic criteria for MS and take in to consideration the clinical presentation, as well

> **Box 3.1 Summary of expected MS findings on MRI**
>
> - Isointense lesions on T1-weighted images
> - Hyperintense lesions on T2-weighted images
> - Lesions are multiple and may be small and punctate or large and confluent
> - Ovoid lesions are called Dawson's fingers
> - Lesions do not normally have mass effect
> - Interface between corpus callosum and septum pellucidum (callosal–septal interface) is common
> - Lesions affect periventricular white matter, corpus callosum, visual pathways, posterior fossa structures and cervical cord
> - Can affect grey matter, but is usually spared
> - Optic neuritis is rarely seen on imaging, but MS eventually develops in 50–70% of patients
> - May be a mass lesion with enhancement (tumoural MS)
> - Acute MS enhances in a pattern that may be nodules, rings or arcs
> - Lesions are dynamic, with changing phases of demyelination, oedema and possibly remyelination. They change shape, size, signal intensity and enhancement of lesions

as CSF, MRI and visual evoked potential findings. The relevant MRI features for diagnosing MS include the number, location and enhancement (on T1-weighted images) of T2 hyperintense plaques.

What are the mimics of MS on MRI?
- Cerebral ischaemia
- Metastases
- Vasculitis
- Encephalitis
- Sarcoidosis
- Post-viral demyelination (acute disseminated encephalomyelitis, ADEM)
- Leucodystrophy

However, helpful features of MS on MRI include: multiplicity of lesions, if >3 mm in diameter with at least one >6 mm, involvement of the corpus callosum and presence of lesions in brainstem, cerebellum or spinal cord.

What other causes of ring enhancing lesions should you consider?
- Common:
  - abscess

- malignant glioma
- intracerebral haematoma (3–6 weeks old)
- lymphoma (especially in transplant patients and in AIDS)
- metastases
- Less common:
  - large aneurysm
  - craniopharyngioma
  - cysticercus cyst
  - tuberculoma
  - atypical meningioma
  - radiation necrosis

What therapeutic options are available for Miss Johnstone?

There is no known cure for MS at present. However, there are promising therapies that may slow the disease. The goal of treatment is to control symptoms and maintain a normal quality of life.

Drugs and other treatments may include:
- Immune modulators to help control the immune system, including interferons and monoclonal antibodies
- Steroids to decrease the severity of attacks when they occur
- Plasma exchange
- Muscle antispasmodics
- Cholinergic medications to reduce urinary problems

- Antidepressants for mood or behaviour symptoms
- Physical therapy, speech therapy, occupational therapy and support groups can help improve the person's outlook, reduce depression, maximize function and improve coping skills

Susan was treated aggressively with immune modulators, steroids and plasma exchange and improved significantly from a clinical perspective. A further MRI study was performed to assess the lesions.

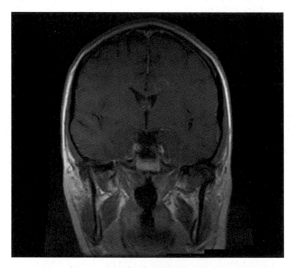

Figure 3.8 Coronal T1-weighted images of the brain following intravenous gadolinium at presentation.

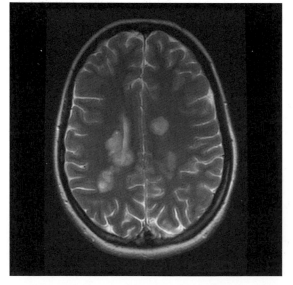

Figure 3.7 Axial T2-weighted image through the brain.

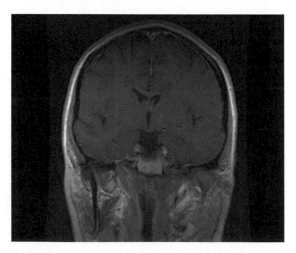

Figure 3.9 Coronal T1-weighted images of the brain following intravenous gadolinium 2 months later.

What do these images show?

After aggressive treatment with immune modulators, steroids and plasma exchange, repeat MRI demonstrated a similar distribution of T2 hyperintense plaques (Fig. 3.7), but no longer with any enhancement after contrast medium administration (Figs 3.8 & 3.9). Appearances suggest a recovery from the active inflammatory demyelination phase seen previously.

What would you expect might be the pattern and course of Susan's disease?

Disease progression, age of onset, gender and prognosis are somewhat characteristic of the four classifications of MS:

1 *Relapsing remitting MS* (RRMS) in 70% of cases. There are clinical exacerbations with clear remission periods, but leaving minimal or no residual sequelae. This typically occurs in females, is of early onset and has the best prognosis. Our patient fits in to this category at presentation.

2 *Primary progressive MS* (PPMS) in 20% of cases. There is chronic disease progression from the onset with an occasional plateau period. The cervical cord is commonly affected and resulting in a myelopathy. This occurs in both males and females, is of later onset and poor prognosis.

3 *Secondary progressive MS.* Starts off as RRMS but with gradual progression of disease. More than 50% of RRMS patients develop this 10 years following onset.

4 *Progressive relapsing MS.* This is unusual, and starts off as PPMS but with subsequent acute relapses with or without full recovery.

PART 2: CASES

CASE REVIEW

Susan Johnstone, a 26-year-old civil servant, presented with a 1 month history of bilateral numbness in hands and feet, fatigue and generalized weakness. She had noticed some blurred vision over the previous 2 weeks. She was referred for a specialist neurological opinion and on further questioning she recalled experiencing similar but milder symptoms during the previous summer.

The clinical diagnosis of MS was suspected and Susan underwent a battery of tests, including an MRI study of the brain and spinal cord. This showed multiple lesions which were hypointense on T1-weighted images, hyperintense on T2-weighted images and exhibited variable enhancement patterns following administration of intravenous gadolinium.

Susan was treated aggressively with immune modulators, steroids and plasma exchange and made a significant improvement clinically. A repeat MRI study showed no change in the T2 appearances, with persistence of multiple hyperintense lesions. However, the lesions were no longer enhancing with intravenous gadolinium, indicating a recovery from the acute inflammatory phase.

KEY POINTS

- MS may present in a number of ways with seemingly unassociated neurological features
- The diagnosis is primarily a clinical one
- Laboratory investigations on the CSF are powerful indicators of MS
- Radiological investigation is almost exclusively with MRI
- Imaging is aimed at identifying typical lesions and excluding other diseases that may mimic symptoms of MS

- The diagnostic criteria for MS take in to account clinical, laboratory and radiological findings
- Following treatment (and recovery) the lesions will persist on T2-weighted images
- Contrast enhanced images allow better evaluation of acute inflammatory and chronic lesions
- There are four patterns of disease in MS, with characteristic demographic patterns and prognosis

Case 4 A 45-year-old woman with weight loss

Jane Askew, a previously well 45-year-old woman, presents to her general practitioner with a 1-month history of drenching night sweats. On further questioning, the patient has unintentionally lost 4 kg in weight recently and feels tired. Physical examination is unremarkable and the patient is referred to the radiology department for a chest radiograph.

What abnormalities are demonstrated on the chest radiograph?

There is a large mass of soft tissue density arising from the mediastinum (Fig. 4.1). The mass is predominantly left-sided, but there is a component on the right side. The mass is obscuring the left heart border superiorly (anterior mediastinum), but the margins of the pulmonary vessels (middle mediastinum) and descending aorta (posterior mediastinum) are clearly seen through the mass. Therefore this is an anterior mediastinal mass. The lungs and pleural spaces are clear. There are no bone or soft tissue abnormalities.

What is the differential diagnosis for these appearances?

- *Lymphadenopathy:*
  - malignancy (lymphoma, carcinoma)
  - infection (particularly tuberculosis)
  - sarcoidosis
- *Thyroid mass:* retrosternal extension is most common with a multinodular goitre
- *Thymic lesion:* a heterogeneous group of tumours which are relatively uncommon
- *Germ cell tumour:* lesions often contain calcification and/or fat, but this may not be visible on the plain X-ray.

Radiology: Clinical Cases Uncovered. By A. S. Shaw, E. M. Godfrey, A. Singh and T. F. Massoud. Published 2009 by Blackwell Publishing. ISBN 978-1-4051-8474-8.

Which of these is most likely?

The anterior mediastinal mass is very bulky, without any extension to the thoracic inlet to suggest it arises from the thyroid gland. The short clinical history suggests an aggressive process; night sweats and weight loss are often seen in patients with lymphoma and tuberculosis. In Western Europe, lymphoma would be the more likely cause of these appearances.

What further radiological investigation would you request?

The patient needs a CT of the neck, chest, abdomen and pelvis to:
- Determine the extent of mediastinal involvement
- Stage the disease
- Identify a suitable site for tissue biopsy (if there are no palpable nodes)

A selection of CT images is presented in Figs 4.2–4.7:

What abnormalities are demonstrated on the CT images?

- Large soft tissue mass in the anterior mediastinum (Fig. 4.3, arrow):
- extending through anterior chest wall (Fig. 4.2)
- compressing the trachea and left main bronchus (Figs 4.2–4.4)
- Pericardial effusion (Fig. 4.5, arrow)
- Left-sided pleural effusion (Fig. 4.2, arrow)
- Bilateral low density adrenal masses (Fig. 4.6, arrow)
- Low attenuation lesion within the right lobe of the liver (Fig. 4.7, arrow)

A biopsy was performed and the histopathologist reported the diagnosis to be diffuse large B-cell lymphoma (DLBCL). This is a high-grade non-Hodgkin lymphoma (NHL).

What stage is the disease?

The lymphomas are staged according to the Ann Arbor classification and Cotswold revision (Box 4.1). The

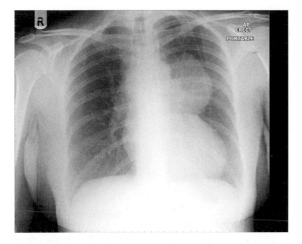

Figure 4.1 PA chest radiograph.

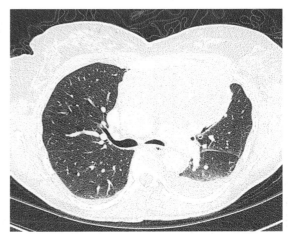

Figure 4.4 Axial CT image (lung windows) at the level of the main bronchi.

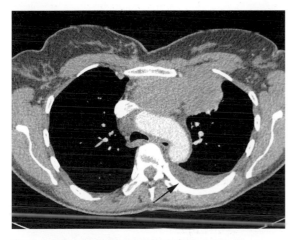

Figure 4.2 Axial CT image at the level of the aortic arch.

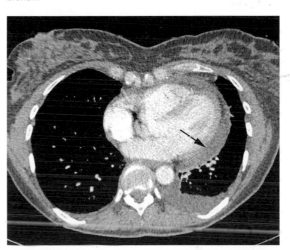

Figure 4.5 Axial CT image at the level of the heart.

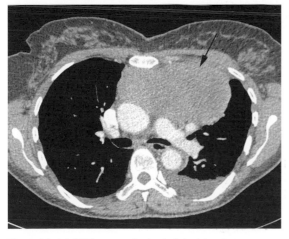

Figure 4.3 Axial CT image at the level of the left pulmonary artery.

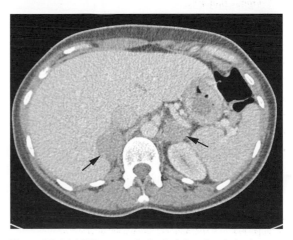

Figure 4.6 Axial CT image at the level of the adrenal glands.

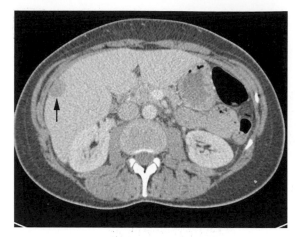

Figure 4.7 Axial CT image at the level of the renal hilum.

presence of multiple extranodal disease sites (liver and adrenal glands) makes this case Stage IV disease. The clinical features are termed 'B symptoms'.

What size is considered 'normal' for lymph nodes identified at CT?

The development of CT technology has enabled clear depiction of smaller and smaller lymph nodes. Measured in the 'short axis', perpendicular to the longest axis of a node in the axial plane, the size considered normal ranges from 6 mm in the retrocrural space to 12 mm in the subcarinal and para-aortic spaces. However, there is a significant degree of overlap between reactive and malignant nodes – small lymph nodes may contain foci of tumour and large nodes may be reactive.

What alternative imaging techniques are available for staging lymphoma?

Positron emission tomography (PET) using 2-[fluorine-18] fluoro-2-deoxy-D-glucose (FDG) provides a 'metabolic map' of the body by mimicking the action of glucose. Cells take up FDG as they would glucose, but cannot metabolize it. The FDG is trapped in the cells and can be detected from its emissions. FDG-PET has consistently been shown to be superior to CT in correctly staging patients with high-grade NHL in addition to Hodgkin's lymphoma. It is of limited value in low-grade disease: the lower metabolic activity of the cells means that FDG is less reliably taken up. Combined PET-CT machines providing both functional and anatomical information have been developed and represent current

---

Box 4.1 Ann Arbor staging classification and Cotswold revision

Stage	Area of involvement
I	A single lymph node region or a single localized involvement of an extralymphatic site
IE	Localized involvement of a single extralymphatic organ or site
II	Two or more lymph node regions on the same side of the diaphragm
IIE	Localized involvement of a single extralymphatic organ or site and of one or more lymph node regions on the same side of the diaphragm
III	Lymph node regions on both sides of the diaphragm
IIIE	Lymph node regions on both sides of the diaphragm accompanied by localized involvement of an extralymphatic organ or site
IV	Diffuse involvement of one or more extranodal organs with or without lymph node involvement
	Localized involvement of a single extralymphatic organ or site with non-regional lymph node involvement

Additional qualifiers

A	Absence of systemic symptoms
B	Presence of systemic symptoms
X	Bulky disease, defined as a nodal mass >10 cm in maximum diameter or mediastinal mass >1/3 of the internal diameter of the thorax on a PA chest radiograph

---

best practice in staging lymphoma. At the moment this is a relatively expensive technique and access is limited in many centres.

Mrs Askew was commenced on multi-agent chemotherapy. Five weeks later she presented to the haemato-oncology team with a cough and breathlessness. The full blood count shows haemoglobin (Hb) 11.7 g/dL, white cell count (WCC) 0.1, platelets (Plt) 47 × 10⁹/L. A chest X-ray was requested.

What does the chest radiograph show?
- Left subclavian venous line *in situ*
- Cavitating lesion in the left upper lobe (projected between fifth and sixth posterior ribs; Fig. 4.8, upper arrow)

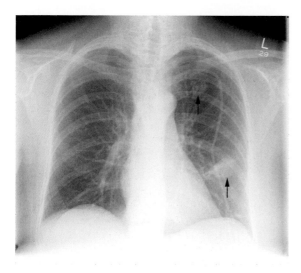

Figure 4.8 PA chest radiograph.

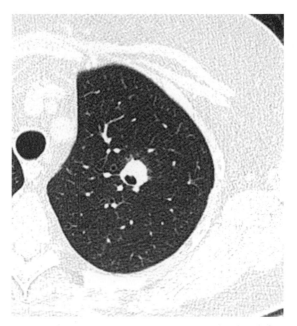

Figure 4.9 Magnified CT image of the left upper lobe.

- Soft tissue lesion in the left mid–lower zone (lower arrow)
- The mediastinal mass appears to have resolved

l *In view of these findings, a CT of the thorax was performed.*

What abnormalities are present?
Left upper lobe (Fig. 4.9):
- Cavitating lesion with a thick wall
- Small halo of ground glass opacification
  Left lower lobe (Fig. 4.10):
- Peripheral wedge-shaped area of consolidation

What is the most likely diagnosis?
Infection is the most likely cause for these appearances in this case. The patient is immunocompromised with a low white cell count. Patients receiving chemotherapy for haematological malignancy are particularly vulnerable to atypical infections; these appearances are typical of fungal infection. The 'halo' of ground glass opacification surrounding lesions is caused by local pulmonary haemorrhage. Cavitation is a sign of central necrotic tissue; this may be present at diagnosis or develop during treatment, where it is a sign of healing.

As the mediastinal disease is improving, new sites of lymphoma in the lungs at this time would be extremely unlikely. Drug reactions may cause pulmonary abnormalities, but not cavitating lesions.

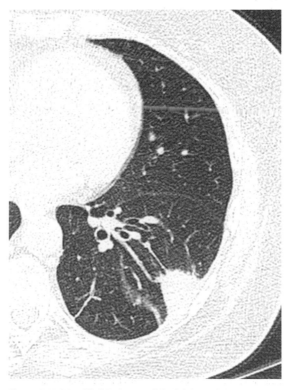

Figure 4.10 Magnified CT image of the left lower lobe.

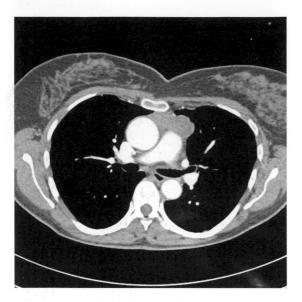

Figure 4.11 Axial CT image at the level of the main pulmonary artery.

A CT-guided biopsy confirmed the diagnosis of angio-invasive aspergillosis and the patient was treated appropriately with antifungal agents. On completion of chemotherapy, Mrs Askew underwent a further CT study to assess response (Fig. 4.11).

What does this image demonstrate?

There is a residual soft tissue mass in the anterior mediastinum. Assuming that all other disease sites have resolved, this represents a partial response to chemotherapy (Box 4.2). Approximately 40% of patients treated for NHL will have a residual soft tissue mass, only 20% of whom will have residual disease.

How might you assess this further?

Percutaneous biopsy of this lesion would be hazardous given its proximity to the aorta and main pulmonary artery. Furthermore, the residual tissue may not be uniform throughout, thus there may be sampling errors. As highlighted above, functional imaging with FDG-PET depicts areas of the body that are metabolically active. In this situation FDG-PET may be helpful in differentiating residual tumour from fibrosis.

> **Box 4.2 International Workshop Criteria for Response Assessment in Lymphoma**
>
> - **Complete response (CR)** Complete disappearance of all detectable disease on CT with previously involved nodes on CT >1.5 cm in their greatest axial diameter regressing to <1.5 cm, and nodes of 1.0–1.5 cm regressing to <1.0 cm. In addition, resolution of disease-related symptoms, normalization of biochemical abnormalities and normal bone marrow biopsy
> - **Complete response unconfirmed (CRu)** Corresponds to CR criteria, but with a residual mass >1.5 cm in greatest axial diameter that has regressed by >75% in the sum of the product of the greatest diameters (SPD)
> - **Partial response (PR)** At least 50% reduction in the SPD of the six largest nodes with no increase in the size of the other nodes and no new sites of disease. Hepatic and splenic nodules should also decrease by at least 50% in the SPD
> - **Stable disease (SD)** Response is less than a PR but is not progressive disease
> - **Progressive disease (PD)** More than 50% increase in the SPD of any previously abnormal node, or appearance of any new lesions during or at the end of therapy
> - **Relapsed disease (RD)** The appearance of any new lesion or increase in size of >50% of previously involved sites or nodes in patients who achieved CR or CRu

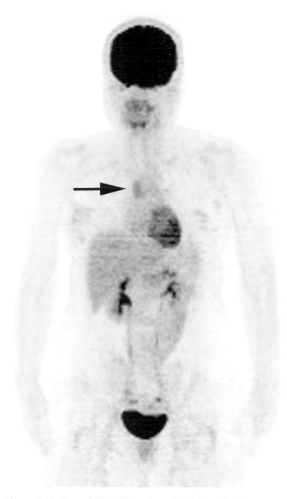

Figure 4.12 Coronal FDG-PET maximum intensity projection image

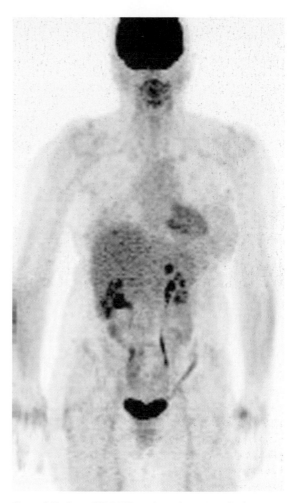

Figure 4.13 Coronal FDG-PET maximum intensity projection image.

What does this image show?

The image shows normal uptake in those tissues that utilize glucose (brain, vocal cords, heart and liver) (Fig. 4.12). There is excretion of FDG seen in the renal tract bilaterally. However, there is abnormal uptake seen in the mediastinum just to the right of midline, indicating the presence of some residual tumour.

Mrs Askew received further chemotherapy but there were no further changes in the CT appearances. A further PET study was requested (Fig. 4.13).

What does this study show?

On this occasion there is a normal distribution of tracer uptake, with no evidence of residual disease. Hence, using the revised response criteria (Box 4.3) Mrs Askew is deemed to have had a complete response to therapy.

Three months later, Mrs Askew represented to the clinical team with vertigo. On examination, there were no lateralizing signs and examination was otherwise unremarkable. A CT of the head was requested (Figs 4.14 & 4.15).

What does the CT study show?

There is a soft tissue density lesion centred on the cerebellar vermis which demonstrates uniform enhancement following administration of intravenous contrast medium.

Box 4.3 Radiological response definitions including FDG-PET

Response	Definition	Nodal masses	Spleen, liver
CR	Disappearance of all evidence of disease	(a) FDG-avid or PET positive prior to therapy; mass of any size permitted if PET negative (b) Variably FDG-avid or PET negative; regression to normal size on CT	Not palpable, nodules disappeared
PR	Regression of measurable disease and no new sites	≥50% decrease in SPD of up to 6 largest dominant masses; no increase in size of other nodes (a) FDG-avid or PET positive prior to therapy; one or more PET positive at previously involved site (b) Variably FDG-avid or PET negative; regression on CT	≥50% decrease in SPD of nodules (for single nodule in greatest transverse diameter); no increase in size of liver or spleen
SD	Failure to attain CR/PR or PD	(a) FDG-avid or PET positive prior to therapy; PET positive at prior sites of disease and no new sites on CT or PET (b) Variably FDG-avid or PET negative; no change in size of previous lesions on CT	
Relapsed disease or PD	Any new lesion or increase by ≥50% of previously involved sites from nadir	Appearance of a new lesion(s) >1.5 cm in any axis, ≥50% increase in SPD of more than one node, or ≥50% increase in longest diameter of a previously identified node >1 cm in short axis Lesions PET positive if FDG-avid lymphoma or PET positive prior to therapy	>50% increase from nadir in the SPD of any previous lesions

What is the diagnosis?

Mrs Askew has relapsed with lymphoma in the cerebellar vermis. Uniform enhancement is typical of lymphoma; infection is usually associated with oedema and a ring-enhancing pattern. A low-grade primary CNS tumour could mimic this, but a high-grade CNS tumour or secondary deposit would also have oedema and ring enhancement.

Mrs Askew was treated with a further course of chemotherapy and then radiotherapy. A subsequent MRI study of the brain confirmed resolution of the cerebellar lesion, but showed abnormalities in the white matter around the lateral ventricles (Fig. 4.16).

What is the likely cause of this?

Periventricular white matter abnormalities are seen more commonly in the ageing population, where they are attributed to small vessel ischaemia. In this instance, with a young patient, these changes are secondary to the micro-vascular ischaemia that occur with cranial radiotherapy.

What symptoms might the patient experience as a consequence?

She may experience mild–moderate cognitive decline, but a focal neurological deficit would be unusual.

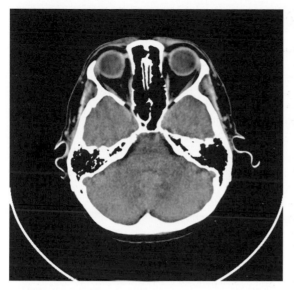

Figure 4.14 Axial CT image through the brain at the level of the cerebellum acquired before administration of intravenous contrast medium.

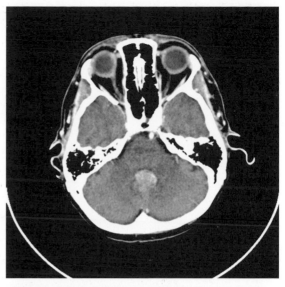

Figure 4.15 Axial CT image through the brain at the level of the cerebellum acquired after administration of intravenous contrast medium.

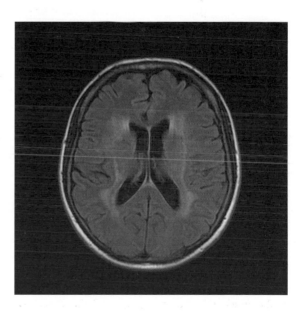

Figure 4.16 Axial FLAIR (T2-weighted with suppression of water signal) image of the brain at the level of the lateral ventricles.

CASE REVIEW

A 45-year-old woman presents to her GP with a short history of night sweats, weight loss and malaise, but normal clinical examination. The clinical symptoms are typical for lymphoma or tuberculosis and the GP requests a chest radiograph which demonstrates a bulky mediastinal mass most consistent with a diagnosis of lymphoma. Cross-sectional imaging and a biopsy are performed to confirm the diagnosis and determine the stage of the disease. On chemotherapy, the patient acquires a chest infection, proven by histology to be fungal.

Following completion of chemotherapy, the CT shows a residual mass in the anterior mediastinum which requires further evaluation. Functional imaging with FDG-PET confirms the presence of residual tumour and further treatment is given. This results in a complete response as judged by a further FDG-PET study.

A few weeks later, the patient develops vertigo and relapse of the lymphoma in the cerebellar vermis is diagnosed on CT imaging. This responds to combined chemotherapy and radiotherapy and once again the patient achieves a complete response. However, the effects of radiotherapy on the periventricular white matter are visible radiologically.

KEY POINTS

- Lymphoma may present with non-specific symptoms
- Drenching night sweats and unintentional weight loss are B symptoms
- The frontal chest radiograph can determine the location of a mediastinal mass to narrow the diagnostic possibilities
- Full staging requires CT (+/− FDG-PET) of the neck, chest, abdomen and pelvis
- Accurate staging allows determination of management and prognosis

- Neutropenic patients are at high risk of atypical infections and these should be managed aggressively
- A residual mass following treatment may be tumour or fibrosis; FDG-PET is needed to differentiate between these
- Relapse of disease may occur at any site, at any time
- Focal neurological signs should be investigated thoroughly, but cognitive decline may be a consequence of cranial radiotherapy

A 47-year-old woman with severe back pain

Anne Johnson presented to her general practitioner complaining of severe pain throughout her spine which had become progressively worse over the past 3 months. In recent days, the pain had begun to radiate down her limbs. Aged 47, Mrs Johnson had no previous medical complaints and there was no history of trauma to account for the back pain. On examination, the spine was tender to palpation at several sites. The general practitioner referred Mrs Johnson for X-rays of the whole spine.

What do these images show?

There is a wedge compression fracture of the L3 vertebral body with approximately 50% loss of anterior vertebral body height (Fig. 5.1). There are several focal areas of lucency within the vertebral bodies. Careful evaluation of this vertebra also reveals that there is loss (destruction) of the normal cortical margin both anteriorly and posteriorly. The L1 and T12 vertebrae also appear abnormal with focal areas of lucency seen. Alignment of the vertebrae is normal, with preservation of the disc spaces between vertebrae.

How would you interpret these findings?

There are a number of potential causes for fractures of the vertebral bodies, with osteoporosis and trauma being the most common. However, such severe changes are unlikely to be brought about by either of these in an otherwise well woman of this age and in the absence of major trauma. Also, neither of these conditions would give lucent lesions nor result in destruction of the normal bony cortex.

The combination of bony destruction and fractures indicates that there is an infiltrative process within the bones. The presence of multiple lesions indicates that this is a disseminated aggressive process. Preservation of the intervertebral disc spaces indicates that this is unlikely to be caused by infection; in the spine, infection is usually centred on the discs rather than the bones. Therefore, the features seen in this image suggest disseminated malignancy.

Which tumours (non-bony) commonly involve bone? How might they appear?

- Metastatic deposits:
  - lung: lytic
  - breast: lytic or mixed lytic and sclerotic
  - renal: lytic lesions, often expansile
  - thyroid: lytic lesions, may be expansile
  - prostate: sclerotic
- Haematological malignancy:
  - myeloma: lytic
  - lymphoma: lytic or sclerotic
  - leukaemia: discrete lesions not usually seen on plain films

Breast examination was normal. Therefore Mrs Johnson had a number of blood tests and was referred for an urgent CT of the chest, abdomen and pelvis to try to identify a primary malignancy and assess the extent of disease. On CT, the lungs and abdominal viscera had normal appearances. A sagittal image of the lumbar spine on bony windows is shown in Fig. 5.2.

Results from the blood tests demonstrated mild anaemia (9 g/dL; normal range 13–17 g/dL) and an elevated corrected serum calcium (13 mg/dL; normal range 8.5–10.2 mg/dL).

What is the most likely diagnosis?

The CT examination has excluded pulmonary and renal malignancy, while breast examination was normal

Radiology: Clinical Cases Uncovered. By A. S. Shaw, E. M. Godfrey, A. Singh and T. F. Massoud. Published 2009 by Blackwell Publishing. ISBN 978-1-4051-8474-8.

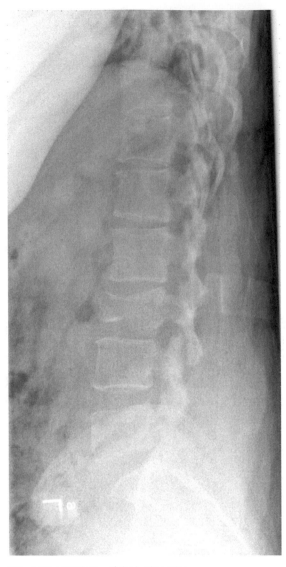

Figure 5.1 Lateral view of the lumbar spine.

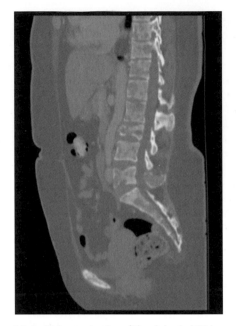

Figure 5.2 Sagittal reconstruction of the abdominal CT images to demonstrate the lumbar spine.

> **Box 5.1 Multiple myeloma**
>
> - Neoplastic proliferation of plasma cells within the bone marrow
> - Usually associated with an abnormal monoclonal protein in the blood or urine
> - Approximately 2800 new cases per annum in the UK
> - Median age is 70 years; fewer than 2% of patients are under 40 years of age
> - May present with signs of bone marrow failure (anaemia or infection), bone pain, fractures, hypercalcaemia, hyperviscosity or fatigue
> - Treatment is primarily with chemotherapy and bone marrow transplantation
> - Treatment is palliative; there is no cure for multiple myeloma

---

(although this does not exclude breast malignancy). Thyroid malignancy often gives metastases to other organs in addition to bone. Of the haematological malignancies, the pattern of disease seen in this case is typical of multiple myeloma (Box 5.1).

Mrs Johnson underwent further blood tests including serum electrophoresis, 24-hour urine collection and bone marrow biopsy. These demonstrated an elevated monoclonal protein within the blood; histopathological analysis of the bone marrow confirmed the marrow was largely replaced with plasma cells, diagnostic of multiple myeloma.

How might you assess the extent of disease in patients with multiple myeloma?

The skeletal survey has been used for many years and is the basis for the majority of evidence in the published literature. The appearance and distribution of lesions on

> **Box 5.2 Radiological appearances of multiple myeloma**
>
> The characteristic bone lesion seen in multiple myeloma is a well-defined small lytic area with no reactive bone formation which arises in the medulla. The absence of bone sclerosis at the margins is because of inhibition of osteoblastic activity. As the lesions grow bigger, they may cause endosteal scalloping (curved lucent indentations on the inner aspect of the bony cortex), then frank cortical destruction and fractures. However, in around 15% of patients, there are no focal lesions, just generalized osteopenia. The most commonly affected sites are the vertebrae (approximately 65% of cases), ribs (45%), skull (40%) and pelvis (30%), whereas the distal bones are rarely involved. Tumour masses (plasmacytomas) may arise from bone or the soft tissues.

> **Box 5.3 Imaging techniques for assessing patients with myeloma**
>
> **Skeletal survey**
> * Plain films of the skull, chest, humeri, femora and pelvis, together with AP and lateral films of the whole spine
> * Readily available
> * Time-consuming to acquire (45 minutes)
> * Lesions are only visible after 30–75% bone loss
>
> **Whole body CT**
> * More sensitive than plain films
> * Higher radiation dose (2–5×, depending on the protocol used)
> * Rapid acquisition (<30 seconds imaging time)
> * Will identify fractures and help predict which bones are at risk of fracture
>
> **Whole body MRI**
> * More sensitive than plain films and CT
> * No radiation
> * Not widely available at present
> * Time-consuming, but newer protocols are reducing examination time
> * Particularly valuable in spinal imaging
>
> **PET (or PET-CT) imaging**
> * Most sensitive test
> * High radiation and cost
> * Very time-consuming
> * Limited availability at present
>
> **Bone scintigraphy**
> * Because of the lack of osteoblastic activity, this is often normal and has no place in multiple myeloma

plain film is described in Box 5.2. Of late, a number of other imaging techniques have been used in patients with multiple myeloma. The main pros and cons of each technique are discussed in Box 5.3.

Mrs Johnson was diagnosed with Stage 3 disease according to the Salmon and Durie classification (Box 5.4). She then underwent a skeletal survey to image those bones not included on the CT study (Figs 5.3 & 5.4).

Why was this felt to be necessary?

There are two main reasons for completing the skeletal survey. The first is to assess those bones not seen on the CT study for critical lesions, i.e. those at risk of progressing to a pathological fracture. Secondly, the images provide a baseline against which any further disease progression may be judged. It is important to bear in mind that CT images of the body are usually acquired with the patient's arms raised above the head.

Do these images raise any concerns?

The skull vault has numerous lytic lesions with a well-defined margin and no sclerotic rim, typical of multiple myeloma but of no consequence in themselves. The proximal (upper) half of the left humerus shows two large areas of lucency, one in the head and another one-third of the way down the bone. There is no evidence of a fracture on this film, but the risk of a fracture needs to be assessed (Box 5.5).

Mrs Johnson reported only a mild ache in the left arm. As the lesion was greater than two-thirds of the diameter of the humerus, a score of 8 was calculated using the fracture risk chart. Therefore Mrs Johnson was referred for radiotherapy for the lesions in the left humerus and commenced on systemic chemotherapy. Three days after starting chemotherapy, Mrs Johnson complains of worsening back pain. Neurological examination found some reduction in power in both legs, but no sensory loss.

What would you do now?

Mrs Johnson has extensive metastatic disease throughout the vertebral column and has developed focal neurological signs. Therefore there should be a high degree of

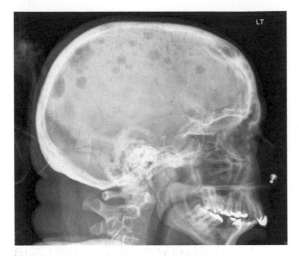

Figure 5.3 Image of the skull from the skeletal survey.

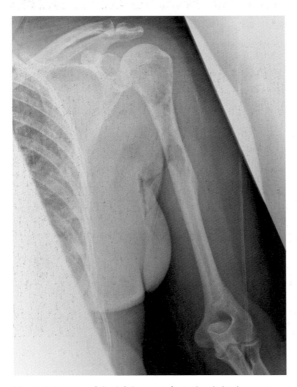

Figure 5.4 Image of the left humerus from the skeletal survey.

suspicion that there is compression of the spinal cord. As such, an urgent MRI of the whole spine should be performed, regardless of whether the signs point to a specific level. Often, multiple (unexpected) foci of tumour may be demonstrated which will significantly affect future management. However, it is always worth

---

Box 5.4 Salmon and Durie staging classification for multiple myeloma

Stage	Criteria
Stage 1	Low tumour mass ($<0.6 \times 10^{12}$ cells/m^2) Haemoglobin >10 g/dL; IgG <5 g/dL, IgA <3 g/dL Bence Jones protein <4 g/24 hour Normal serum calcium level Normal or solitary bone lesion
Stage 2	Intermediate tumour mass (0.6–1.2 $\times$ 10^{12} cells/m^2) Haemoglobin, IgG, IgA, Bence Jones protein and serum calcium ranges between Stage 1 and 3 levels
Stage 3	High tumour mass ($>1.2 \times 10^{12}$ cells/m^2) Haemoglobin <8.5 g/dL; IgG >7 g/dL; IgA >5 g/dL Bence Jones protein >12 g/24 hour Serum calcium level >12 mg/dL (adjusted for albumin) Advanced lytic bone lesions

---

Box 5.5 Scoring system for diagnosing impending pathological fractures

Variable	Score		
	1	**2**	**3**
Site	Upper limb	Lower limb	Peritrochanteric
Pain	Mild	Moderate	Functional
Lesion	Blastic	Mixed	Lytic
Size	<1/3 diameter	1/3–2/3 diameter	>2/3 diameter

- A score of 7 or less (5% probability of fracture) suggests a low probability of fracture, such that conservative management (chemotherapy and/or radiotherapy) is appropriate
- A score of 8 (15% probability of fracture) is highly suggestive of impending fracture. In this situation, the relative benefits of surgery need to be weighed against the risk of fracture in the individual patient
- A score of 9 or more (33% probability of fracture) is diagnostic of impending fracture; this is an indication for prophylactic fixation of the bone

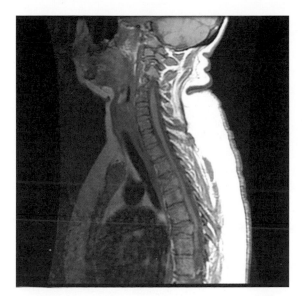

Figure 5.5 Sagittal T1-weighted image through the cervical and thoracic spine.

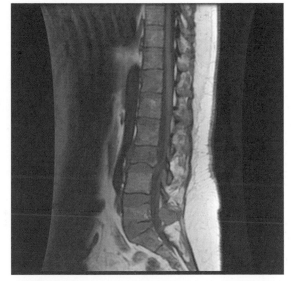

Figure 5.7 Sagittal T1-weighted image through the thoracic and lumbar spine.

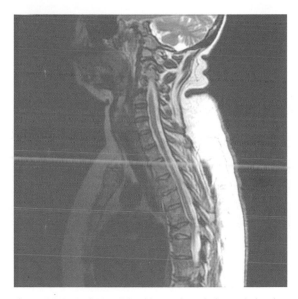

Figure 5.6 Sagittal T2-weighted image through the cervical and thoracic spine.

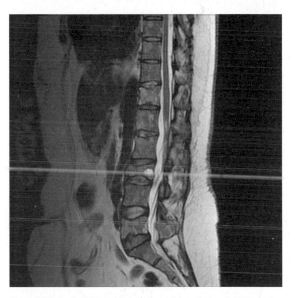

Figure 5.8 Sagittal T2-weighted image through the thoracic and lumbar spine.

indicating the expected site of disease as the radiographer can start imaging at that location; patients with severe back pain may not tolerate the full examination and it is crucial to image key areas first (Figs 5.5–5.8).

What do these images demonstrate?

Normal imaging of the bone marrow is essentially similar to fat, because this is found in significant quantities in normal marrow. Thus, on T1-weighted images, the bone marrow should return a higher signal than the adjacent discs, and on T2-weighted images should return a lower signal. On both sequences, the signal should be relatively homogeneous.

On these images, the signal within the vertebral bodies is heterogeneous throughout the spinal column with vertebral body fractures seen in the mid-thoracic as well as

---

Box 5.6 MRI features of benign and malignant vertebral body fractures

	Benign fracture	**Malignant fracture**
Marrow signal	Band of low signal adjacent to fracture (acute)	Diffuse low signal on T1-weighted images
	Normal on all sequences (old fracture) Normal signal preserved opposite the fractured end plate	High or heterogeneous signal on T2-weighted images Round or irregular foci of marrow replacement Posterior elements involved Soft tissues or epidural involvement
Contrast enhancement	Homogeneous 'return to normal' signal after injection	High or heterogeneous signal
Vertebral contours	Retropulsion of a posterior bone fragment (often postero-superior)	Convex posterior cortex

---

the lumbar region. There is further abnormal signal which can be seen in the posterior elements at L5. This reflects diffuse marrow involvement with tumour. The fractured vertebrae protrude in to the canal, with the thoracic fracture pressing on the spinal cord. However, CSF can be seen behind the cord indicating that there is no cord compression. Remember that the spinal cord terminates at L1, hence the L3 lesion cannot cause cord compression. It may cause pressure on or irritation of the lumbar nerve roots.

The key features that help differentiate benign from malignant fractures on MRI are listed in Box 5.6.

Mrs Johnson is discharged home and remains well for several months. At an outpatient clinic, she is told that the abnormal protein levels have reduced and that she has had a partial response to her therapy. She asks whether she should have an X-ray to check whether the bone lesions have resolved.

What should you request?

Nothing should be requested at this stage. Bony lesions seldom improve with therapy, and when they do it is a process that takes many months if not years. If the patient is otherwise well, progress should be monitored through blood tests primarily.

One year later, Mrs Johnson attends clinic and tells you that she has had some pain in her left hip over the past few days. Blood tests are performed and an X-ray of the pelvis is carried out.

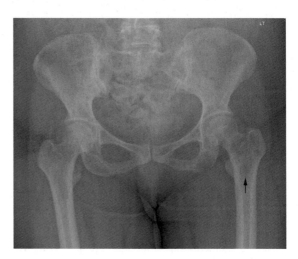

Figure 5.9 AP view of the pelvis.

What does the image show?

There is a large ill-defined lucent lesion in the intertrochanteric region of the left hip (Fig. 5.9, arrow). In addition, there are a number of smaller lesions seen in both proximal femora with scalloping of the bony cortex.

The earlier images are reviewed and these lesions were not present. A CT of the hip is requested to establish the extent of disease in the left hip.

What does the CT image show?

On the left of Fig. 5.10, the image demonstrates a lytic lesion greater than two-thirds of the diameter of the

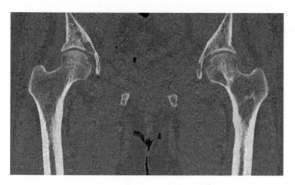

Figure 5.10 Coronal reconstruction of the left hip CT images.

cortex in a peritrochanteric position. However, on the right side there is just a little osteopenia and no discrete focal lesion is evident.

What would you do now?

Using the scoring system from Box 5.5, this is at high risk for fracture and an orthopaedic opinion should be sought with regard to internal fixation.

Mrs Johnson underwent surgical fixation of the left femoral neck. Blood tests confirmed disease progression with a rise in serum protein. Mrs Johnson's chemotherapy regime was altered and she was referred for consideration of bone marrow transplantation.

CASE REVIEW

Anne Johnson is a 47-year-old woman with a 3-month history of progressively worsening back pain. In the days before presenting to her GP, the pain had become more pronounced and was beginning to radiate down her legs. Her GP requested plain films of the lumbar spine which demonstrated multiple lucent lesions and a wedge compression fracture of the L3 vertebral body suggestive of malignancy.

Imaging with CT demonstrated widespread lytic bone lesions, but the lungs and abdominal viscera were found to be normal. Serum electrophoresis and bone marrow biopsy confirmed the diagnosis of multiple myeloma. A skeletal survey was performed which identified lytic lesions in the left humerus at risk of fracture; these were treated with radiotherapy.

Mrs Johnson developed further back pain and abnormal neurological signs. An MRI of the whole spine was performed which demonstrated diffuse malignant disease throughout the bone marrow and several fractured vertebrae. However, there was no evidence of cord compression.

Mrs Johnson initially had a good response to chemotherapy but later complains of pain in the left hip. A pelvic radiograph and subsequent CT demonstrate a new large lytic lesion at the left hip considered to be at high risk of fracture. She was referred for surgical fixation of this hip.

Disease progression was confirmed by elevated serum proteins and Mrs Johnson was considered for further therapy.

KEY POINTS

- Multiple myeloma usually presents in patients over 40 years of age
- It may present with symptoms of bone marrow failure, bone pain or non-specific systemic symptoms
- The diagnosis is made by demonstrating an abnormal monoclonal protein on serum electrophoresis, 24-hour urine collection or bone marrow sampling
- Staging of patients with multiple myeloma is usually performed with a skeletal survey
- Typically, myeloma lesions are lucent with no sclerotic rim
- Vertebral body fractures are commonly seen in patients

with myeloma; they may result from malignancy or bone demineralization
- CT and MRI may be helpful in evaluating focal bone lesions at risk of fracture and other potential complications such as spinal cord compression
- Bone lesions at high risk of fracture may be treated by radiotherapy or surgical fixation
- Treatment for multiple myeloma is based on chemotherapy and bone marrow transplantation
- The aim is to prolong survival and reduce complications but is essentially palliative; there is no cure as yet

Case 6 An 11-month-old boy with abdominal pain

Joseph Holt, an 11-month-old boy, presents with his mother to his GP for an urgent appointment. She describes how that morning, for a short period, his eyes were 'jerking around wildly' and that his legs appeared to be twitching. Mrs Holt wondered whether Joseph had had a 'fit' and whether she should take him to the hospital. When asked about Joseph's general well-being, his mother told the GP that her son had intermittent 'colicky' abdominal pain for the past 2 weeks, but that she had thought this might be caused by constipation.

Review of the medical notes revealed that Joseph had been born at full term with a normal delivery. There were no other medical problems, his development had been normal to this stage and he was not taking any medication.

The GP examines Joseph's abdomen and finds a hard mass in the right upper quadrant which seems to be slightly tender. Examination was felt to be otherwise unremarkable.

What is the differential diagnosis for a right upper quadrant mass in a child?

The differential diagnosis is wide and best approached on an organ-by-organ basis:

- Liver:
  - hepatomegaly (acute hepatitis, congenital liver disease)
  - hepatic tumour (primary, either benign or malignant; metastases)
- Kidney:
  - hydronephrosis (secondary to renal tract obstruction)
  - Wilms' tumour (most common tumour in children)
  - cystic renal disease

Radiology: Clinical Cases Uncovered. By A. S. Shaw, E. M. Godfrey, A. Singh and T. F. Massoud. Published 2009 by Blackwell Publishing. ISBN 978-1-4051-8474-8.

- Adrenal gland:
  - neuroblastoma
- Bowel:
  - constipation
  - intussusception (usually presents with acute abdominal pain and often associated with blood-stained faeces described as like 'redcurrant jelly')
- Lymph nodes:
  - lymphoma

The GP refers Joseph urgently to the local hospital, where he is seen by the paediatrician. He confirms the examination findings of the GP, and also notes that his blood pressure is elevated. The paediatrician obtains blood and urine samples from the little boy and arranges imaging of his abdomen.

What investigations would you request at this stage and why?

- Blood samples:
  - full blood count – to assess for evidence of infection and bone marrow function
  - urea and electrolytes – to assess renal function
  - liver function tests – to assess hepatic function
  - glucose – deranged glucose metabolism per se may cause seizures; adrenal pathology is one of the causes of abnormal glucose metabolism
- Urine sample:
  - microscopy – to check for haematuria, tumour cells and infection
  - biochemistry – to check for vanillylmandelic acid (VMA) or homovanillic acid (HVA), catecholamines secreted by neuroblastoma that are excreted in urine
- Imaging:
  - ultrasound of the abdomen – to confirm the presence of a mass and, if present, to try and establish the organ of origin. There is no ionizing radiation involved and no sedation will be required to obtain the images

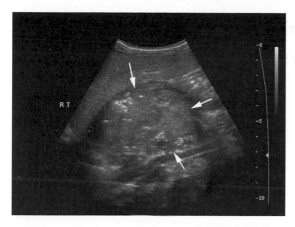

Figure 6.1 Longitudinal ultrasound image in the centre of the abdomen.

What does the ultrasound image show?

There is a large heterogeneous abdominal tumour mass lying posterior to the liver and anterior to the aorta (Fig. 6.1, arrows).

The ultrasound report also states that the liver, spleen and kidneys appear normal.

What is the next stage of the patient's management?

A CT study of the chest, abdomen and pelvis to determine the origin and extent of tumour. A child of this age will need to be sedated for this procedure to avoid movement artefacts.

What do the CT images show?

• There is a large mass centred on the right side of the abdomen (Fig. 6.2, arrows)
• This mass lies posterior to the liver and antero-superior to the right kidney
• There are punctate areas of calcification within the mass
• There is displacement of the liver, kidneys and blood vessels by the mass
• There are soft tissue density nodules seen in the subcutaneous tissues (Fig. 6.3, arrows)

On review of the laboratory results, the urinary VMA levels are elevated, but the blood tests are all within normal limits.

What is the diagnosis?

The patient has a neuroblastoma (Box 6.1).

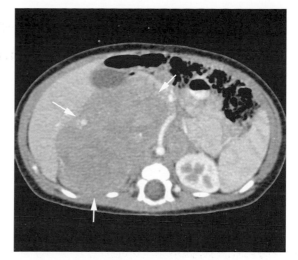

Figure 6.2 CT image through the abdomen at the level of the spleen following administration of intravenous contrast medium.

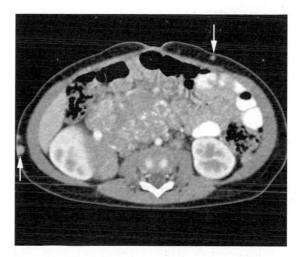

Figure 6.3 CT image through the abdomen at the level of the kidneys following administration of intravenous contrast medium.

Box 6.1 Neuroblastoma

• Tumours arise from the neural crest
• Fewer than 100 cases/year in the UK (incidence 1 in 10,000)
• Most common solid abdominal tumour in infancy
• Second most common tumour in childhood (Wilms' tumour is more common in older children)
• Peak age at presentation is 2 years; 25% <1 year
• Equal sex incidence

Box 6.2 Associations and presentation of neuroblastoma

General
- Pain
- Fever
- Limp/off legs

Neurological
- Cerebellar ataxia
- Proptosis

Catecholamine production
- Hypertension
- Diarrhoea
- Encephalopathy
- Flushing and/or sweating
- Hyperthermia
- Hyperglycaemia

Box 6.3 International Neuroblastoma Staging System

Stage 1	Localized tumour with complete gross excision, with or without microscopic residual disease
Stage 2A	Localized tumour with incomplete gross excision
Stage 2B	Localized tumour with or without complete gross excision, with ipsilateral non-adherent lymph nodes positive for tumour
Stage 3	Unresectable unilateral tumour infiltrating across the midline
Stage 4	Any primary tumour with dissemination to distant lymph nodes, bone, bone marrow, liver, skin and/or other organs, except as defined for Stage 4S
Stage 4S	Localized primary tumour, as defined for Stage 1, 2A or 2B, with dissemination limited to skin, liver and/or bone marrow (limited to infants younger than 1 year)

How does this diagnosis explain all of the patient's symptoms and signs?

- *Eye movements and leg twitching:* opsoclonus–myoclonus is an uncommon but characteristic presentation of neuroblastoma; it occurs in about 2–3% of children with the tumour. It is also known as 'dancing eyes, dancing feet', which describes the involuntary movements of the eyes and legs during attacks. It is thought to be a paraneoplastic phenomenon
- *Elevated blood pressure:* present in 30% of cases, this is caused by increased production of catecholamines by the neuroblastoma

See Box 6.2 for other associations and presenting symptoms.

What further imaging investigation(s) is required to complete staging?

^{131}I-metaiodobenzylguanidine scan

This study involves the injection of a radioactive isotope of iodine labelled with ^{131}I-metaiodobenzylguanidine (MIBG). Uptake occurs in amine precursor and decarboxylase (APUD) tumours that originate from neural crest cells and synthesize catecholamines. This study enables non-invasive evaluation of the extent of bone marrow involvement. If the tumour does take up ^{131}I-MIBG then a much higher dose may be given as part of the patient's therapy (Fig. 6.4).

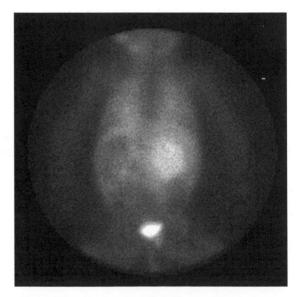

Figure 6.4 Posterior view of an ^{131}I-MIBG scan. This demonstrates uptake in the right upper quadrant, but no evidence of distant disease.

This test is also used in other APUD tumours (phaeochromocytoma, medullary thyroid carcinoma, carcinoid tumour).

Bone marrow biopsy

To assess bone marrow involvement in patients with advanced disease.

MRI of the spine

This should be performed if the tumour is in the paraspinal region to assess whether it has extended through the neural foramina.

How is neuroblastoma staged?

Neuroblastoma is staged according to the International Neuroblastoma Staging System (Box 6.3).

How does this relate to prognosis?

The prognosis for patients with neuroblastoma is a combination of tumour stage, the age of the patient and the tumour biology. Increasing stage and age >1 year worsen prognosis.

However, Stage 4S neuroblastoma is unusual in having an approximately 80% survival rate (compared with 7% for Stage 4).

What treatment is available for neuroblastoma?

- Surgery – for localized tumours
- Chemotherapy – for unresectable and/or metastatic disease
- Radiotherapy – external beam radiotherapy or radioactive ^{131}I-MIBG for disseminated disease

CASE REVIEW

Joseph, an 11-month-old boy, is brought to his GP for an urgent appointment with unusual neurological signs. Careful questioning raises questions about non-specific abdominal symptoms, and on examination he is found to have an abdominal mass and hypertension. In the first instance, an ultrasound of the abdomen is used because it is safe and enables a thorough examination of the abdomen in children. Using this in combination with simple blood and urine tests, the diagnosis of neuroblastoma may be confirmed and other conditions systematically excluded.

Having made a diagnosis of malignancy, the patient needs complete staging of his tumour in order that therapy can be planned and the prognosis determined. Clearly, for optimal patient management, a multidisciplinary approach is required involving paediatrician, oncologist, surgeon, pathologist and radiologist.

KEY POINTS

- Children often present with non-specific signs and symptoms
- Parental concerns should not be dismissed lightly
- A thorough clinical examination is essential, even of apparently unconnected systems
- Childhood tumours are relatively uncommon, but if suspected need urgent and thorough investigation
- When imaging children, particular care must be taken to avoid any unnecessary ionizing radiation; ultrasound is ideal in this respect
- Cross-sectional imaging of young children will often require some form of sedation
- The management of tumours in childhood is undertaken by specialist clinical teams in dedicated centres

Case 7 A 10-year-old boy with a painful arm

Philip Jones, a 10-year-old schoolboy, presents to his GP with his mother. He complains of a painful right arm which has been getting progressively worse. As a consequence, Mrs Jones reports that Philip has not been sleeping very well recently, particularly the last 3 weeks. He often walks in to his parents' room in the middle of the night holding his right arm complaining of a dull ache. On occasions he also says that his arm is painful to touch.

What are the important points to cover in Philip's history?

It is important when assessing children to take a full medical and social history, covering everything from birth problems, immunization history and social background. Somatic symptoms can sometimes indicate psychological problems.

However in this case, the key features are as follows:

- Onset:
  - can a precipitant be identified?
- Description of the pain:
  - what is it like?
  - where is it precisely?
  - when does it occur?
  - what makes it better?
  - what makes it worse?
- Previous episodes:
  - have there been any associated features?
  - are any other sites involved?
  - does anything else occur with the pain?
- Social history:
  - sports activities
  - school difficulties, e.g. bullying
  - always remember non-accidental injury, although unusual at this age

---

Radiology: Clinical Cases Uncovered. By A. S. Shaw, E. M. Godfrey, A. Singh and T. F. Massoud. Published 2009 by Blackwell Publishing. ISBN 978-1-4051-8474-8.

Philip tells the GP that he cannot recall any bumps or injuries to his right arm and cannot pinpoint exactly when the pain started. He tells him that it has come on gradually over the last few weeks and reiterates that it seems much worse at night and is concentrated solely in his right arm. His mother tells him that they have given Philip some paracetamol without effect, but that ibuprofen seemed to ease the pain somewhat. They tell him this has never happened before. It transpires that Philip is a keen sportsman, playing cricket and tennis almost every day as it is the summer.

On physical examination Philip was asked to point to where his pain occurs. He points to the upper aspect of his right arm over the biceps muscle, and finds it slightly tender when the GP palpates this region. No other abnormality was found on examination and Philip does not seem to be in any distress as the GP talks to him.

What are the potential causes of Philip's symptoms?

- Trauma:
  - sport-related injury
  - undisclosed injury to the arm
  - non-accidental injury
- Focal bone lesion:
  - benign
  - malignant
  - infective
- Soft tissue lesion
- Systemic illness:
  - haematological malignancy

What would be your initial management steps?

The clinical history is very non-specific. There do not seem to be any features of systemic illness or significant trauma and there is no mass to feel. The fact that the pain seems worse at night and is relieved by non-steroidal anti-inflammatory drugs (NSAIDs) is typical of many

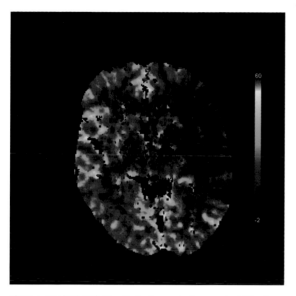

Plate 1 Cerebral perfusion study demonstrating cerebral blood flow.

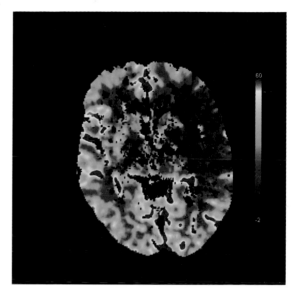

Plate 2 Cerebral perfusion study demonstrating cerebral blood volume.

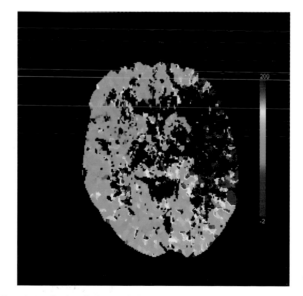

Plate 3 Cerebral perfusion study demonstrating time to peak enhancement.

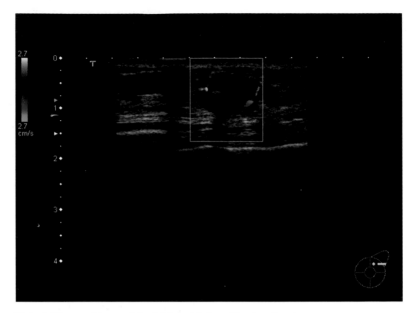

Plate 4 Ultrasound image of the left breast lesion with colour Doppler.

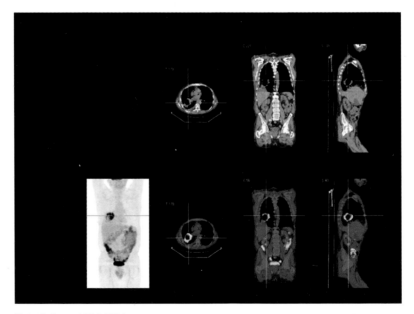

Plate 5 Coronal FDG-PET image.

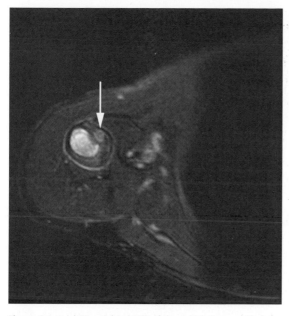

Figure 7.1 Axial T2-weighted MRI of the right humerus with fat saturation.

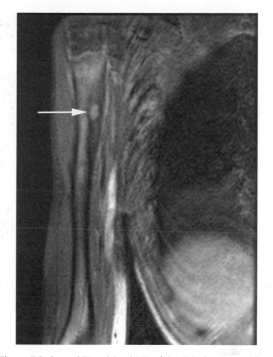

Figure 7.2 Coronal T1-weighted MRI of the right humerus with fat saturation.

musculoskeletal complaints. It is most likely that the pain is related to his sporting activities.

> Philip's GP prescribed some more NSAIDs for Philip and advised him to rest from his sporting activities for a few weeks. Philip's mother said that she had read on the Internet that MRI was very good in the assessment of sports injuries. Under pressure from Philip's mother, the GP agreed to refer Philip for an MRI to try to ascertain the cause of the problem.

What imaging should the GP have requested?

When faced with a patient who complains of musculoskeletal pain in the appendicular skeleton for which there is no obvious cause, the plain film should always be the starting point for imaging.

Describe the MR images

The humerus can be seen centrally on the axial image with normal high signal from the bone marrow. Within the surrounding low signal bony cortex, there is a small focus of high signal. The cortex also appears to be a little thicker medially than laterally. The coronal T1-weighted image shows the lesion in the medial aspect of the right

humerus within the bony cortex. The muscles appear normal. The lesion has been highlighted with arrows (Figs 7.1 & 7.2).

> The radiologist reports the presence of a focal bone lesion in the cortex of the right humerus and advises that a plain film be performed to help characterize the lesion further (Figs 7.3 & 7.4).

What are the key features when describing a focal lucent lesion within bone?

One of the most important features to note is the patient's age. Some lesions, e.g. solitary bone cyst, are very rarely seen over the age of 30 years. The key features of the actual lesion are listed in Box 7.1.

What does this film show?

Within the upper third of the right humerus (within the diaphysis) there is a small focal lucent lesion with a well-defined sclerotic margin. There is no calcification within the matrix of the lesion, but there does appear to be some thickening of the cortex medially which may be reactive. There is no periosteal reaction or cortical disruption.

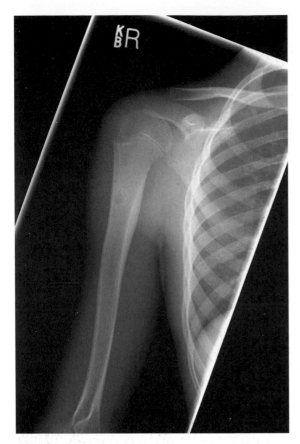

Figure 7.3 AP radiograph of the right humerus.

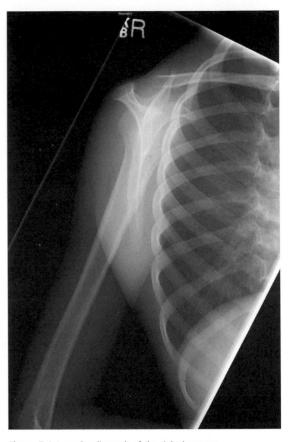

Figure 7.4 Lateral radiograph of the right humerus.

> **Box 7.1 Features to assess when evaluating focal lucent bone lesions on plain films**
>
> - Size
> - Site
>   ○ Epiphysis, metaphysis or diaphysis
>   ○ Cortex or medulla
> - Margin
>   ○ Sharp or ill-defined
> - Matrix
>   ○ Calcification?
> - Reaction
>   ○ Periosteal reaction?
>   ○ Reactive sclerosis?
>   ○ Is the cortex intact?
> - Soft tissues
>   ○ Is there soft tissue extension?

What are the potential causes of a well-defined lucent lesion in the bone of such a young patient?

- Solitary bone cyst:
  ○ unilocular, does not cause reactive sclerosis
- Non-ossifying fibroma:
  ○ painless, does not cause reactive sclerosis
- Aneurysmal bone cyst:
  ○ large expansile lesion
- Chondroblastoma:
  ○ epiphyseal location
- Osteoid osteoma
- Infection
- Eosinophilic granuloma

The plain film has helped to narrow down the differential diagnosis significantly to osteoid osteoma, infection and eosinophilic granuloma. The latter is less likely to cause symptoms and also less likely to be sited within the cortex. Philip's blood tests were normal other than a mildly raised C-reactive protein (CRP) of 12.

Box 7.2 Osteoid osteoma

- Benign bone lesion
- Aetiology unknown
- Most common in the second decade
- Uncommon in patients >30 years of age
- Affects males twice as often as females
- Accounts for approximately 10% of benign bone tumours
- Most common location is the femur, followed by the tibia, posterior elements of the spine, and the humerus
- Clinical picture of dull pain that is worse at night and disappears within 20–30 minutes of treatment with NSAIDs
- Local symptoms can include an increase in skin temperature, increased sweating and tenderness
- Epiphyseal lesions can cause abnormal growth
- Spinal lesions may cause scoliosis

What further imaging might be of value?

Bone scintigraphy would likely be positive in all of these conditions. However, it would be of value if multiple lesions were suspected in order to aid detection.

A CT of the right humerus would be helpful to try and narrow the differential diagnosis further by getting a clear image of the bone.

Philip was referred for a CT examination of his right humerus (Figs 7.5 & 7.6).

What do the CT images show?

There is a small lucent lesion within the bony cortex. This does not contain any calcification. There is marked thickening of the cortex adjacent to the lesion caused by reactive sclerosis. There is no disruption of the cortex.

What is the most likely diagnosis?

The radiological features on plain film and CT are typical of an osteoid osteoma (Box 7.2) but similar features may also be seen in osteomyelitis. However, the MRI showed that this central lucent nidus was a vascularized structure with enhancement following intravenous gadolinium. Osteomyelitis would have an avascular purulent nidus. If the MRI study had not already been performed, then bone scintigraphy could also be used to show this feature.

What treatment options are available?

An osteoid osteoma will typically resolve spontaneously in 2–4 years, hence it may be left alone and the patient

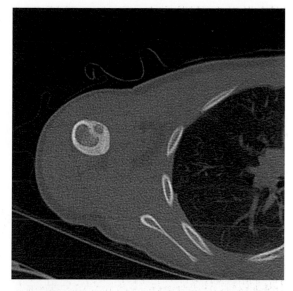

Figure 7.5 Axial CT image of the right humerus on bone windows.

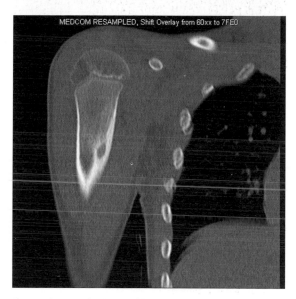

MEDCOM RESAMPLED, Shift Overlay from 60xx to 7FE0

Figure 7.6 Coronal CT image of the right humerus on bone windows.

given analgesia. However, many patients do not wish to stay on analgesics and there are two methods of treatment:

1 *Percutaneous ablation:* using image guidance and a radiofrequency probe
2 *Surgical resection:* the nidus is resected en bloc

Philip opted for surgical resection, with complete resolution of his symptoms.

CASE REVIEW

A 10-year-old schoolboy, Philip Jones, presents with a 3-week history of pain in the right arm, worse at night. There is no obvious precipitant for the pain, but he seems to obtain relief from NSAIDs. The clinician suspects a sports-related injury and refers Philip for an MRI of the right humerus. A focal lesion is noted on the MRI with uptake of gadolinium.

Further assessment of the lesion with plain film imaging and subsequently with CT enabled the diagnosis of an osteoid osteoma to be made. Following a discussion with the orthopaedic team, Philip underwent surgical resection of the nidus and made a full recovery.

KEY POINTS

- Musculoskeletal symptoms are common and usually non-specific
- Initial imaging of unexplained musculoskeletal pain in the appendicular skeleton should be with plain films
- There are many different types of focal bone lesion and the plain film is very useful in diagnosis or guiding further imaging
- If an abnormality is detected, or symptoms persist, further imaging with CT, MRI or bone scintigraphy should be performed
- Osteoid osteoma is a common benign bone lesion that causes pain and may lead to skeletal deformity
- It will spontaneously resolve in time, but many patients do not wish to remain in pain over a long period and opt for resection or percutaneous ablation

A 48-year-old woman with a breast lump

Mary Greene, a 48-year-old teacher, presents with a right-sided breast lump she noticed when in the shower. She goes to see her GP who refers her to the local breast unit for triple assessment.

What are the three components of triple assessment?

The three components of triple assessment are:

1 Clinical examination
2 Radiology (either ultrasound, mammography, MRI or a combination of these)
3 Pathology (either cytology or, more often, histology)

On arrival at the breast unit, the patient is seen by the breast surgeon who takes her history and examines her.

What are the important questions to ask?

Box 8.1 gives the relevant questions to ask a patient with a breast lump. The responses from the patient were as follows:

Presenting complaint. Lump in right breast.
History of presenting complaint. The lump was first noticed 1 week ago and is not painful. Mrs Greene has not noticed any skin changes or nipple discharge. She has not found any other lumps elsewhere.
Past medical history. The patient had a breast cyst aspirated when she was 40. She started her periods aged 13 and has not gone through the menopause.
Drug history. She has never used hormone replacement therapy but took the oral contraceptive pill for about 5 years starting in her early twenties.

Radiology: Clinical Cases Uncovered. By A. S. Shaw, E. M. Godfrey, A. Singh and T. F. Massoud. Published 2009 by Blackwell Publishing. ISBN 978-1-4051-8474-8.

Family history. Her maternal aunt had breast cancer at 55. No family history of ovarian cancer.
Social history. Two children, the first born when she was 27, both of whom were breastfed for 6 months.

As such, Mrs Greene is not considered to be at high risk for breast cancer. Nevertheless, breast cancer is the most common cancer in the UK, with women having a 1 in 9 chance of developing it at some stage of their life.

Why are these questions important?

Aside from the questions about the lump, most of these questions relate to the patient's lifelong oestrogen exposure. This is an important risk factor for breast cancer. An increase in exposure, e.g. caused by an early menarche, will increase the risk of breast cancer.

Women are asked about ovarian problems because of the *BRCA1* and *BRCA2* genes, both of which significantly increase the risk of breast and ovarian cancer. *BRCA2* is also often implicated in cases of breast cancer in men.

What are the key features to assess in the examination?

Box 8.2 gives the important points to note during breast examination.

Mrs Greene has a 2-cm lump in the upper outer quadrant of the right breast. It is firm in consistency and not fixed to the underlying tissues. There are no palpable axillary or supraclavicular lymph nodes.

How would these examination findings be scored?

Given the lump's relatively small size, consistency and lack of fixity/associated lymphadenopathy, this lump would be rated as E2 clinically, or benign (Box 8.3).

Box 8.1 History relevant to breast disease

Presenting complaint. What has the patient noticed?

History of presenting complaint. Lump: how long for, pain associated with it, skin changes, nipple discharge, lumps elsewhere (other breast or lymph nodes)?

Past medical history. Previous lumps, previous breast imaging or surgery? Age at menarche and menopause (if applicable)

Drug history. Has the patient ever taken hormone replacement therapy or the oral contraceptive pill?

Family history. Any blood relatives with breast or ovarian problems?

Social history. Any children? If so were they breastfed? Mother's age at birth of first child?

Box 8.2 Key features of breast examination

- Skin changes (peau d'orange, nipple inversion, Paget's disease of the breast, erythema)
- Size of lump
- Consistency of lump
- Fixity of the lump to the skin or underlying tissues
- Are there any enlarged axillary or supraclavicular lymph nodes?

Box 8.3 Clinical examination scoring

E1 Normal
E2 Benign
E3 Indeterminate, probably benign
E4 Indeterminate, probably malignant
E5 Malignant

How would you decide whether to use mammography, ultrasound or MRI for imaging Mrs Greene?

Mammography is used in symptomatic women over the age of 35. Women younger than this have denser breasts (i.e. they contain more glandular soft tissue and less fat). A soft tissue density tumour may go undetected against this background of normal soft tissue. As women age, glandular tissue is progressively replaced by fat, against which a soft tissue density tumour will be more easily identified.

Box 8.4 National Institute for Clinical Excellence (NICE) guidelines for patients suitable for yearly breast magnetic resonance screening

- *BRCA1* or *BRCA2* carriers aged 30–49 years
- P53 mutation carriers over 20 years
- Age 30–39 years:
  - No known mutation but a 10-year risk of greater than 8%
- Age 40–49 years:
  - No known mutation but a 10-year risk of greater than 20%
  - No known mutation but a 10-year risk of greater than 12% with a dense pattern on plain film mammography

A patient's 10-year risk is calculated using their family history, e.g. two close relatives diagnosed with breast cancer at an average age of less than 30 constitutes an 8% 10-year risk in a 30- to 39-year-old

---

Mammograms are always compared with any previous imaging. In Mrs Greene's case, she would not have started having screening mammograms. In the UK, women are invited to undergo breast screening every 3 years with plain film mammography from the age of 50 to 69 years. In the near future, the programme will be expanded to include all those 47–73 years of age. Any new soft tissue density areas or microcalcification would be considered suspicious.

Breast ultrasound is used whenever there is a palpable lump. Ultrasound images are helpful in guiding diagnosis, and may be used to guide aspiration or biopsy.

MRI is not currently used in routine breast imaging. For the majority of patients, mammography and ultrasound are sufficient to obtain a diagnosis. However, current guidelines recommend the use of breast MRI to screen for tumours in young women with a high risk of breast cancer. This has the advantage of not exposing the patient to ionizing radiation, as well as being more sensitive than plain film mammography. The patients eligible for yearly screening with breast MRI are listed in Box 8.4. In the UK, breast MRI outside these high-risk patients is currently restricted to problem-solving (e.g. in those patients with breast implants) and research programmes.

I *Mrs Greene has bilateral mammograms (Figs 8.1–8.4).*

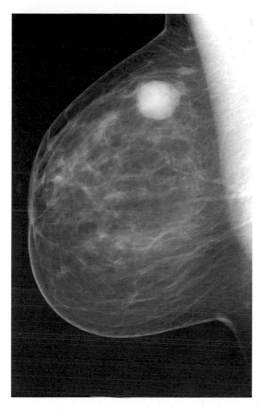

Figure 8.1 Mediolateral oblique mammogram of the right breast.

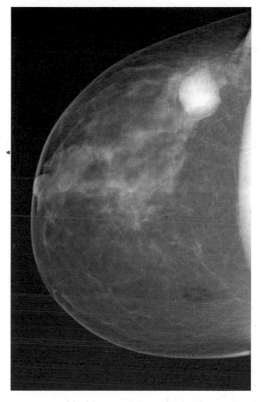

Figure 8.2 Craniocaudal mammogram of the right breast.

Do the mammograms correspond to the history?

Yes, there is a 2-cm soft tissue density mass in the right upper outer quadrant.

In general, what features would suggest malignancy on a mammogram?

A breast neoplasm is more likely if there are any of the following on mammography:

- Microcalcification
- A spiculate mass
- Distortion of the normal breast architecture

What is the differential diagnosis for these appearances?

The lesion in the right breast does not demonstrate microcalcification or spiculation. It has a smooth, rounded, well-defined edge. There is no associated distortion of the normal breast architecture. The appearances suggest a benign lesion, possibly a cyst. A

fibroadenoma (a benign breast lesion) is also possible, but would be more common in younger women.

Is there another abnormality?

Yes, there is another soft tissue mass in the left breast, also in the upper outer quadrant. This mass is more concerning, as it demonstrates microcalcification and has a spiculated margin. The patient was unaware of the mass at presentation, i.e. this mass is not symptomatic.

How would these mammographic appearances be scored?

The rating system for radiological tests is similar to that for clinical examination, as shown in Box 8.5. In this case the right mammogram would be scored as R3, probably benign. The left mammogram would be scored as R5, as it is almost certainly malignant.

The patient is then seen by the radiologist who again clinically examines the patient. In Mrs Greene's case this is

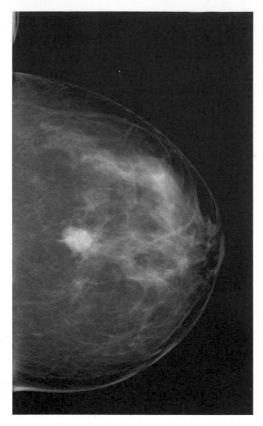

Figure 8.3 Craniocaudal mammogram of the left breast.

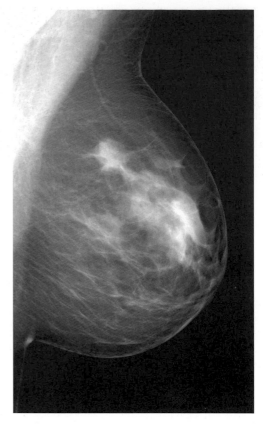

Figure 8.4 Mediolateral oblique mammogram of the left breast.

> **Box 8.5 Radiological scoring**
>
> R1 Normal
> R2 Benign
> R3 Indeterminate, probably benign
> R4 Indeterminate, probably malignant
> R5 Malignant

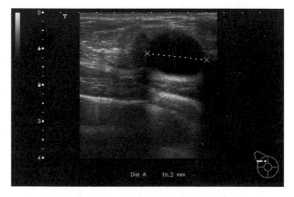

Figure 8.5 Ultrasound image of the right breast lesions.

particularly relevant given the finding of an additional mass on plain film mammography. In retrospect, the lesion in the left breast is also just palpable, although this was missed at the initial clinical examination. The radiologist then performs an ultrasound examination. No enlarged axillary lymph nodes can be found on ultrasound (Figs 8.5 & 8.6).

What do the images show?

In the right breast, there is a 16-mm cyst. In the left, a 12-mm irregular hypoechoic soft tissue mass showing increased blood flow on colour Doppler imaging is seen (Plate 4).

Does this help with the diagnosis?

The lesion in the right breast is definitely a simple cyst: it is thin walled and anechoic (i.e. there are no internal echoes).

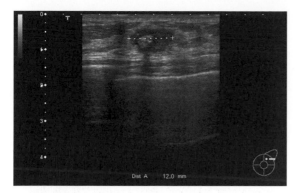

Figure 8.6 Ultrasound image of the left breast lesions.

The ultrasound appearance of the left breast is not diagnostic. In this scenario, pathology is required almost regardless of ultrasound appearances; any hypoechoic palpable lump needs to have a biopsy in order to confirm the pathology.

How would the ultrasound be scored?

The right breast lesion is definitely benign and would be scored as R2. In patients who are symptomatic, ultrasound-guided therapeutic aspiration is offered.

The appearance of the left breast would be scored as R4. There are no features that are diagnostic of malignancy (e.g. invasion of the skin) but the irregular border and increased blood flow are concerning.

The radiologist takes a core needle biopsy of the left breast lump.

Which is better: fine needle aspiration cytology or core needle biopsy?

Each has its advantages and disadvantages. Fine needle aspiration cytology (FNAC) is less invasive than core needle biopsy but only provides information about cellular appearance. Core needle biopsy is slightly more invasive and requires local anaesthetic. However, the solid tissue provides information about cellular appearance and tissue architecture. This allows the pathologist to look for invasion, the hallmark of malignancy.

In recent years there has been a trend away from FNAC towards core needle biopsy. This is for two main reasons: first, there has been a reduction in the size of core biopsy needles making them very well-tolerated by patients. The second reason has been the recognition that many patients undergoing FNAC were requiring a biopsy at a later date because the cellular appearances were indeterminate.

> **Box 8.6 Cytological scoring**
>
> C1 Insufficient sample
> C2 Benign
> C3 Atypical
> C4 Suspicious
> C5 Malignant

> **Box 8.7 Histological types and frequency of primary breast tumours**
>
> | | |
> |---|---|
> | Ductal carcinoma/ductal carcinoma *in situ* | 75% |
> | Lobular carcinoma | 12% |
> | Tubular carcinoma | 8% |
> | Mucinous carcinoma | 2% |
> | Medullary carcinoma | 2% |
> | Papillary carcinoma | 1% |

How is each technique performed?

To perform FNAC the radiologist uses a syringe and 22 g needle. While continuously aspirating, several passes are made through the lesion under ultrasound guidance. The cells obtained are then smeared on a slide and air fixed.

Core needle biopsy is also performed under ultrasound guidance. After local anaesthetic is injected, a small cut (2–3 mm) is made in the skin. A mechanical device propels first a cutting needle and then a sheath through the lesion, obtaining a core of tissue. This is then fixed in formalin, and later processed onto slides for the histopathologist to examine.

Mrs Greene was given the results of the imaging and asked to return in a few days for the results of the biopsy.

How are the results of pathology tests scored?

Cytology is scored in a slightly different way to clinical examination and radiological tests, as shown in Box 8.6.

A core biopsy is not given a score as interpretation is clear-cut: the sample is either benign, or shows evidence of invasion (i.e. demonstrates malignancy). In rare equivocal cases, the biopsy will usually be repeated.

At the follow-up appointment, Mrs Greene was given the result of her biopsy, which shows a grade II invasive ductal carcinoma (Box 8.7). She talks to the surgeon about treatment options and together they plan a wide local excision with a sentinel node biopsy.

What is the sentinel node and how is it identified?

The sentinel node is the first in the chain of lymph nodes draining the tumour. If the sentinel node is clear of tumour, it is assumed that the nodes beyond are also clear. Rather than surgically removing all lymph nodes from the axilla, often the sentinel node alone is excised. If it is free of tumour no further surgery is required. If it is not, a further operation to clear the axilla of nodes may be undertaken. This strategy has reduced rates of complications such as lymphoedema of the arm.

The sentinel node is located by injecting blue dye and/ or a radioactive tracer in to the breast and then looking for it intra-operatively either by sight or with a Geiger counter, depending on the technique used.

Mrs Greene made an uneventful recovery from surgery. The axillary lymph nodes were not involved and this was considered Stage I disease (Box 8.8) and as such has an approximately 90% 5-year survival. Mrs Greene remains on regular surveillance.

Box 8.8 **Staging of primary breast tumours**	
Stage	**Description**
0	Carcinoma *in situ*
I	Tumour does not involve axillary lymph nodes
IIA	Tumour 2–5 cm, node negative, or tumour <2 cm and node positive
IIB	Tumour >5 cm, node negative, or tumour 2–5 cm and node positive (<4 axillary nodes)
IIIA	Tumour >5 cm, node positive, or tumour 2–5 cm with 4 or more axillary nodes
IIIB	Tumour has penetrated chest wall or skin, and may have spread to <10 axillary nodes
IIIC	Tumour has >10 axillary nodes, 1 or more supraclavicular, infraclavicular or internal mammary nodes
IV	Distant metastasis

CASE REVIEW

Mary Greene, a 48-year-old teacher, presents with a lump in the upper outer quadrant of the right breast and is referred for triple assessment at her local breast unit. The lump is firm, smooth and mobile and is therefore clinically considered to be benign. The patient undergoes bilateral mammograms and the lesion again has benign features. However, the mammogram detects a lesion in the left breast which has more sinister features.

With this information, Mrs Greene was then examined by the radiologist and a small mass corresponding to the radiographic abnormality was palpated in the left breast. The radiologist performs an ultrasound examination. The right breast lesion is diagnosed as a simple cyst and the patient is therefore offered ultrasound-guided therapeutic aspiration. The left breast lesion is hypoechoic and irregular, and therefore a core biopsy was performed under ultrasound guidance. No enlarged axillary lymph nodes were identified using ultrasound.

Mrs Greene returned a few days later to be given the histology results of the left breast lesion: a Grade II invasive ductal carcinoma. After discussing the management options with a breast surgeon, they opt for a wide local excision with sentinel node biopsy.

KEY POINTS

- Breast screening is for asymptomatic patients only
- All symptomatic patients should be referred for triple assessment
- Triple assessment comprises:
  - Clinical history and examination
  - Radiology
  - Pathological assessment (usually core needle biopsy)
- For some lesions, mammography and ultrasound are sufficient to exclude the possibility of malignancy (such as with simple cysts)
- For most palpable lesions that are solid on ultrasound, core biopsy is necessary
- Breast MRI is used primarily for young patients at high risk of developing breast cancer

Further reading

Britton P, Sinnatamby R. (2007) Rational imaging: investigation of suspected breast cancer. *BMJ* **335**, 347–8.

Case 9 — A 70-year-old man with haemoptysis

Simon Etkind, a 70-year-old man, presents to his GP with a 1-month history of cough with occasional haemoptysis. On direct questioning he mentions that he has been short of breath recently. He denies having had fevers or sweats, or losing any weight. In terms of past medical history, he had a coronary artery bypass graft (CABG) 4 years ago. He used to smoke 20 cigarettes per day, but gave up when he had his CABG.

On examination the GP notes the midline sternotomy scar, but cardiac examination was otherwise normal. On auscultation there are a few crepitations at both lung bases, but nothing else of note. The patient's temperature is 37.8°C.

What is the differential diagnosis for haemoptysis?

Haemoptysis is a concerning symptom – the important diagnoses to exclude are malignancy and infection (particularly tuberculosis). Most patients will not have these. The differential diagnosis includes the following.

- Infections:
  - bronchitis
  - pneumonia
  - *Mycobacterium tuberculosis*
  - lung abscess
- Neoplasia:
  - primary or secondary lung malignancy
- Vascular:
  - pulmonary embolism
  - arteriovenous malformation (often associated with Osler–Weber–Rendu syndrome (also known as hereditary haemorrhagic telangiectasia)

- Autoimmune:
  - vasculitides (e.g. Wegener's granulomatosis, rheumatoid lung, systemic lupus erythematosus)
  - Goodpasture's syndrome
- Trauma:
  - post intubation
  - foreign body
- Other:
  - bronchiectasis
  - pulmonary oedema
  - bleeding diatheses

What blood tests would you arrange?

- Full blood count – to look for evidence of infection or low platelets
- Urea and electrolytes – as a baseline test for renal function
- Liver function tests – in disseminated malignancy these may be abnormal
- Clotting – to look for a bleeding diathesis
- C-reactive protein (CRP) – for evidence of infection

Is imaging required at this point?

Yes. The patient should be referred for an urgent chest X-ray to try to establish the diagnosis (Fig. 9.1). Early diagnosis may have implications from both a personal and from a public health perspective (on diagnosing TB, everyone who has been in contact with the patient will need to be screened for the disease).

What does the image show?

In the lower zone of the right lung there is a ring-shaped soft tissue density, within which is an air–fluid level. These appearances occur when there is a cavitating lesion in the lung. The hilar structures appear normal. There is no significant volume loss on the right, i.e. the mediastinum is not shifted to the right, nor is the hemidiaphragm raised on that side. There is no pleural effusion.

Radiology: Clinical Cases Uncovered. By A. S. Shaw, E. M. Godfrey, A. Singh and T. F. Massoud. Published 2009 by Blackwell Publishing. ISBN 978-1-4051-8474-8.

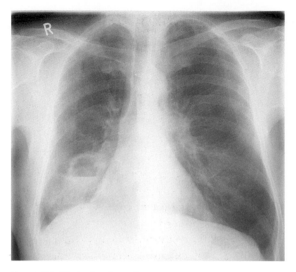

Figure 9.1 PA chest radiograph.

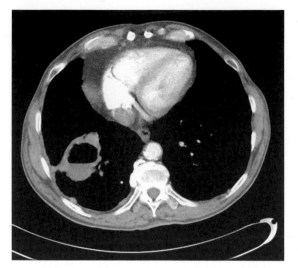

Figure 9.2 Axial CT image of the thorax.

Incidentally, sternal wires can be seen projected in the midline, indicative of previous sternotomy (in this patient's case by CABG).

What is the differential diagnosis for these appearances?

A cavitating lung lesion has a number of potential causes:
- Infection:
  - *Mycobacterium tuberculosis*
  - *Staphylococcus aureus*
  - Gram-negative bacteria, e.g. *Klebsiella pneumoniae*
- Neoplasia:
  - primary malignancy
  - secondary malignancy (especially squamous cell carcinoma)
- Vascular:
  - pulmonary embolism with infarction
  - septic pulmonary emboli
- Autoimmune:
  - Wegener's granulomatosis
- Trauma:
  - pulmonary contusion

A useful mnemonic is CAVITY: Cancer Autoimmune Vascular Infection Trauma Young people (in whom one also needs to consider pulmonary sequestration and duplication cysts).

The blood tests are all normal apart from a raised white cell count (12.1 × 10⁹/L (normal range 4–11)) and CRP 35 mg/L (normal <5).

Are there any other tests that you would consider at this point?

In an elderly ex-smoker with no risk factors (e.g. immunosuppression or known exposure to tuberculosis), malignancy would be the most likely cause at this point. However, given the history of haemoptysis, coupled with a solitary cavitating lesion on the chest radiograph, other causes (particularly infective) should be excluded. In the first instance, have sputum samples sent to microbiology to look for acid-fast bacilli. A tuberculin skin test may also be performed.

A CT examination of the chest and upper abdomen would be the usual next step. This would be useful in:
- Further characterizing the cavitating lesion
- Determining if there are other lung lesions that are too small to see on the chest radiograph
- Determining if there are any enlarged lymph nodes in the axillae, hila or mediastinum
- Assessing the liver for possible metastases
- To guide bronchoscopy

A CT examination of the chest and upper abdomen was performed (Figs 9.2 & 9.3).

The two images are through the same level, why do they look so different? What do they show?

A CT machine produces images made up of a large number of picture elements (pixels). These represent a

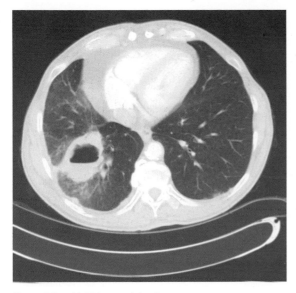

Figure 9.3 Axial CT image of the thorax.

small volume of body tissue (voxel) and are assigned a value in Hounsfield units (HU) according to the average density of material within that voxel compared with water. 0 HU is arbitrarily defined as the density of water, −1000 is air and bone is typically around 1000. Fat has a density less than water, but many of the soft tissues of the body lie between 30 and 70 HU. The eye is able to discern only about 80 shades of grey. To overcome this mismatch, images can be displayed in a variety of different 'windows' that optimize the display for viewing of different tissues. The first image is displayed using a standard soft tissue window, designed for viewing the mediastinum. The second image is displayed using the lung window, which enables the lung parenchyma to be seen in more detail.

The images show the cavitating lesion, again with a fluid level. The lesion has a relatively thick, irregular wall. This would be more suggestive of malignancy than infection. The lesion extends out to the edge of the lung.

On the rest of the CT, there were no enlarged nodes in the axillae, hila or mediastinum, and the liver was free of focal lesions.

How would you take this further?
To characterize the lesion, a biopsy would be needed. Biopsy of lung lesions may be performed under image guidance (usually with CT), or at bronchoscopy. In general, central lesions (i.e. near the hilum) are more suited to bronchoscopic biopsy and peripheral lesions are more suited to image-guided biopsy.

> **Box 9.1 Histological subtypes of lung cancer**
>
> - Non-small cell lung cancer (80%)
>   - Squamous cell carcinoma (30%)
>   - Adenocarcinoma (25%)
>   - Large cell carcinoma (10%)
>   - Bronchoalveolar carcinoma (5%)
>   - Other (10%)
> - Small cell lung cancer (20%)

Mr Etkind underwent bronchoscopy. A biopsy of the lesion was taken and, at the same time, washings were taken and sent for microbiological analysis to look for acid-fast bacilli or other infections.

The biopsy showed squamous cell carcinoma. No acid-fast bacilli or other infective organisms were found. The tuberculin skin test was also negative.

How are lung cancers classified histologically?
Lung cancers are classified in to two main groups:

1 Non-small cell lung cancer (80% of cases)
2 Small cell lung cancer (20% of cases)

This classification is useful because the two groups have very different treatments and prognoses. Non-small cell lung cancer (NSLC) comprises a number of different histological subtypes – the full list is given in Box 9.1.

What further investigations are needed at this point?
Mr Etkind needs to have more accurate staging of his tumour in order to decide whether the disease is amenable to surgical resection. See Box 9.2 for lung cancer staging.

Surgery is offered to patients with Stage 1 or 2 disease. Of crucial importance is determining whether mediastinal nodes are involved. CT can determine whether nodes are enlarged, but cannot differentiate malignant from reactive nodes. If CT is used as the only test of mediastinal lymph node involvement, it results in many unnecessary operations. More recently, FDG-PET or PET-CT has been used in this context. The advantage of PET/PET-CT is that it shows the metabolic activity of cells within a lymph node, rather than relying on changes in lymph node size. It is much more sensitive for detecting early lymph node involvement than cross-sectional imaging (Plate 5).

Box 9.2 Non-small cell lung cancer staging

Stage	Description
T1	<3 cm in diameter, surrounded by lung or visceral pleura
T2	>3 cm in diameter *or* invasion of visceral pleura *or* lobar atelectasis *or* obstructive pneumonitis – at least 2 cm from the carina
T3	Tumour of any size, <2 cm from carina *or* invasion of parietal pleura, chest wall, diaphragm, mediastinal pleura, pericardium *or* pleural effusion *or* satellite nodule in same lobe
T4	Invasion of the oesophagus, vertebral body, carina or a malignant pleural effusion
N0	No involved lymph nodes
N1	Peribronchial *or* ipsilateral hilar nodes
N2	Ipsilateral mediastinal nodes
N3	Contralateral hilar *or* mediastinal *or* scalene *or* supraclavicular nodes
M0	No metastases
M1	Distant metastases
IA	T1, N0, M0
IB	T2, N0, M0
IIA	T1, N1, M0
IIB	T2, N1, M0 *or* T3, N0, M0
IIIA	T3, N1/2, M0
IIIB	T4, any N *or* any T, N3
IV	M1 disease

Is the tumour suitable for surgical resection?

The PET study demonstrates FDG uptake in the lung lesion. There is also normal physiological uptake in the brain and solid abdominal viscera. Of note, there is no

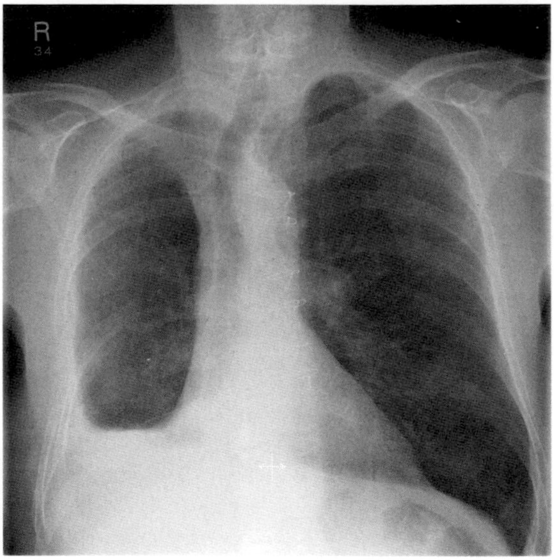

Figure 9.4 PA chest radiograph.

avid uptake in the mediastinum which would indicate lymph node involvement. There are no radiological bars to surgery, but the patient will need an assessment to ensure that he is otherwise fit for the procedure.

Mr Etkind attends outpatient clinic 6 weeks later with the chest X-ray shown in Fig. 9.4.

What does the image show?

There is significant reduction in the volume of the right hemithorax – the mediastinum is shifted to the right. There is a right pleural effusion. No focal lung lesion is seen. There are normal lung markings seen in the right upper zone. The patient has had a right lower lobectomy.

CASE REVIEW

A 70-year-old man presents to his GP with a 1-month history of cough, haemoptysis and shortness of breath. He is an ex-smoker with a past history of CABG. An urgent chest X-ray demonstrates a cavitating lung lesion. The most concerning differential diagnoses at this point are malignancy and infection.

The cavitating lung lesion is further characterized with a CT examination of the chest and upper abdomen. The thick wall is suggestive of carcinoma. No enlarged lymph nodes or distant metastases are identified. Bronchoscopic biopsy confirms the lesion to be a primary squamous cell carcinoma. No evidence of infection is found.

An FDG-PET study is used to accurately stage the disease. There is no nodal disease or distant metastasis. The patient therefore underwent potentially curative surgery.

KEY POINTS

- Haemoptysis is a symptom that should be investigated promptly
- Most patients with haemoptysis will have a benign cause
- Tuberculosis and carcinoma need to be excluded in patients with haemoptysis
- Cavitating lung lesions have a wide differential diagnosis; the clinical context and medical history are crucial in reaching a diagnosis
- Cavitating lung lesions seen on chest X-ray should be further characterized with a CT examination of the chest and upper abdomen

- Biopsy of lung lesions may be performed under image guidance or at bronchoscopy
- Peripheral lesions are more suited to image guided biopsy while central lesions are more suited to bronchoscopic biopsy
- CT is good for T (tumour) staging in lung cancer. It is less sensitive for the detection of involved lymph nodes and distant metastases
- PET or PET-CT enables more accurate staging of N (nodal) and M (metastases) prior to surgery

PART 2: CASES

Case 10 A 31-year-old woman with shortness of breath

Helen Theakston, a 31-year-old woman, presents to the accident and emergency department with a history of sudden onset shortness of breath. In view of the symptoms, the attending physician assesses her initially before taking her history:

Airway	*Helen is talking, but cannot complete sentences*
Breathing	*Respiratory rate is 24 breaths/minute, trachea central*
Circulation	*Pulse 92 beats/minute, regular*
	Blood pressure 110/70 mmHg
	Apex beat not displaced

Pulse oximetry reveals blood oxygen saturation to be 92%, which improves to 99% with 24% oxygen via a Venturi mask. Given the normal position of the trachea and apex beat, the physician rules out a tension pneumothorax.

What is the differential diagnosis for sudden onset breathlessness in a young adult?

- Asthma
- Pulmonary embolism
- Pneumothorax
- Airway obstruction (e.g. inhaled foreign body)
- Drugs (inhaled or injected)
- Anaphylaxis
- Cardiac event (arrhythmia)
- Panic attack – of all the possible causes, this may be ruled out immediately as panic attacks will not result in decreased oxygen saturations

What are the key questions to ask when taking the clinical history?

- Are there any other symptoms?
- Were there any obvious precipitating causes?

Radiology: Clinical Cases Uncovered. By A. S. Shaw, E. M. Godfrey, A. Singh and T. F. Massoud. Published 2009 by Blackwell Publishing. ISBN 978-1-4051-8474-8.

- Has this happened before?
- Is there a history of any respiratory disease?
- Does the patient have any other medical conditions?
- Is the patient on any medication?
- Does the patient have known allergies?
- Does the patient smoke?

What are the key features of the clinical examination?

- Cardiac – is there any evidence of cardiac aetiology or compromise?
- Respiratory – is there any evidence of wheeze (bronchospasm), stridor (upper airway obstruction) or pneumothorax?
- Are the legs swollen (deep vein thrombosis)?

Helen reported that she had some mild central chest pain which did not radiate. There was no history of respiratory illness, smoking, obvious precipitants or allergies. She did have epilepsy, which was well controlled and there had been no changes in her medication recently.

Further to the initial assessment, on examination there were reduced breath sounds and hyper-resonance to percussion on one side. At this stage, Helen was referred for a chest X-ray (Fig. 10.1).

What does the chest X-ray show?

There is a right-sided pneumothorax. The edge of the lung can be seen parallel to the chest wall. Importantly, this confirms the clinical findings that there is no evidence of a tension pneumothorax (central trachea, heart is in the correct position).

A pneumothorax may be categorized according to size as:
- Small: <2 cm between the lung edge and chest wall on chest X-ray
- Large: 22 cm between the lung edge and chest wall on chest X-ray

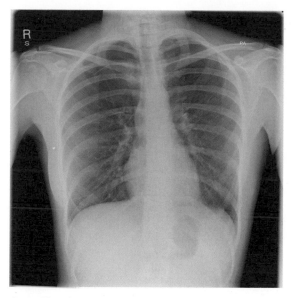

Figure 10.1 Chest X-ray.

Estimation of the precise size of a three-dimensional pneumothorax from the two-dimensional chest X-ray is almost impossible. However, as a rule of thumb, a 1-cm rim of air around the lung equates to approximately 25% of the volume of the hemithorax, while a 2-cm rim is roughly 50%.

The underlying lungs are of normal volume, but the parenchyma is diffusely abnormal. Hence, the pneumothorax is considered to be a secondary pneumothorax (i.e. a pneumothorax in someone with an underlying pulmonary abnormality). Characterization of diffuse lung disease from a chest X-ray alone is difficult, but should begin with identifying the underlying pattern:

- Nodular – predominantly nodules
- Reticular – predominantly lines
- Cystic – thin-walled, air filled, predominantly circular structures

In this case, the pattern is that of cysts.

Would an expiratory chest X-ray be useful?

A chest X-ray taken in expiration increases the conspicuity of a pneumothorax. However, British Thoracic Society (BTS) guidelines stipulate that expiratory films are not recommended for the routine diagnosis of non-traumatic pneumothorax. The diagnosis in this case has already been made so an expiratory film would not be contributory to patient management but would expose her to ionizing radiation.

How would you treat the pneumothorax?

The patient was treated with aspiration, as the pneumothorax was small (<2 cm) and the patient was under 50 years old. The patient was admitted under the care of a respiratory physician. The BTS guidelines for the treatment of pneumothorax are summarized in Fig. 10.2.

What further investigations are needed?

The diffuse lung abnormality depicted on the chest X-ray needs to be further characterized and should prompt further referral and investigation. A high resolution CT (HRCT) of the thorax is indicated to further assess the parenchymal abnormality. A helical (volume) CT may also be of value in the assessment of patients with a persistent pneumothorax. Box 10.1 summarizes the differences between HRCT and standard CT of the chest. Pulmonary function tests will provide information on the effects of the disease process, but should be reserved until the patient recovers from the acute episode.

Why is it called HRCT?

HRCT uses a high spatial resolution reconstruction algorithm. This means that the spatial resolution (or ability to see small details) is maximized at the expense of increasing the noise (manifested as randomly placed dots throughout the image). It is useful in the imaging of lungs because the structures being imaged are small but have very different densities (air versus soft tissue). This is different to the structures in the abdomen where there are relatively smaller differences in density. Figure 10.3 shows an image from the HRCT study.

What does the HRCT image show?

The HRCT confirms the right-sided pneumothorax, and demonstrates the presence of numerous abnormal air spaces within the lungs. These are pulmonary cysts, because they have a perceptible wall. This distinguishes them from emphysematous bullae, which do not have a perceptible wall.

What is the differential diagnosis for this appearance?

- Langerhans cell histiocytosis
- Lymphangioleiomyomatosis
- Neurofibromatosis

Langerhans cell histiocytosis in adults is almost always associated with smoking. The CT appearances are

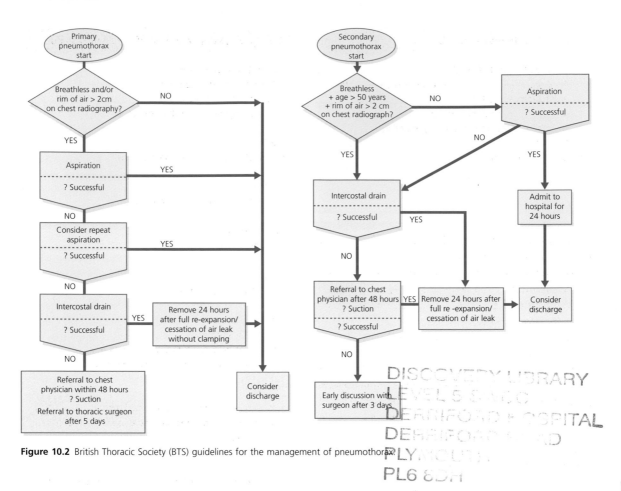

Figure 10.2 British Thoracic Society (BTS) guidelines for the management of pneumothorax.

Box 10.1 **High resolution CT (HRCT) and helical CT**		
	HRCT	**Helical CT**
What does it do?	'Samples' the lung	Images the whole lung
Images	1 mm slice every 10 mm	Contiguous slices
Dose	1 mSv	6 mSv
Good for	Parenchymal diseases	Tumours, vasculature

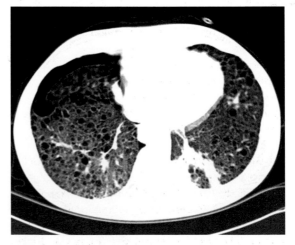

Figure 10.3 Axial CT image through the lower thorax.

> **Box 10.2 Tuberous sclerosis**
>
> - 1 in 5000 to 1 in 10,000 births
> - Mutations of either *TSC1* gene (chromosome 9) or *TSC2* gene (chromosome 16)
> - Autosomal dominant inheritance
> - 60–70% of cases are sporadic, representing new mutations
> - Variable expression

> **Box 10.3 'Major features' of tuberous sclerosis**
>
> **Central nervous system**
> - Cortical hamartomas (tuber)
> - Subependymal nodule
> - Subependymal giant cell astrocytoma
>
> **Ocular**
> - Multiple retinal nodular hamartomas
>
> **Cardiac**
> - Cardiac rhabdomyoma, single or multiple
>
> **Respiratory**
> - Lymphangioleiomyomatosis
>
> **Renal**
> - Renal angiomyolipomas
>
> **Skin**
> - Facial angiofibromas
> - Shagreen patches/connective tissue naevus
> - Hypomelanotic macules/ash-leaf spots (>3)
>
> **Other**
> - Non-traumatic ungal or periungal fibroma
>   Definitive diagnosis requires the presence of two or more of these features.

typically those of nodules which develop in to cysts, which often have bizarre shapes.

Lymphangioleiomyomatosis is a disorder of smooth muscle proliferation in the lungs. In its sporadic form it occurs exclusively in women. It may also be associated with tuberous sclerosis.

Neurofibromatosis gives predominantly apical cysts and is associated with NF-1.

Other causes for cysts are associated with dilated airways (cystic bronchiectasis), fibrosis, consolidation (infection) or septal thickening (lymphocytic interstitial pneumonitis). These are not present in this case.

The clinical team note Helen has several facial lesions, which are confirmed by a dermatologist to be facial angiofibromas.

What is the diagnosis?

Facial angiofibromas is almost pathognomonic of tuberous sclerosis (Box 10.2). The various clinical manifestations of tuberous sclerosis are listed in Box 10.3.

In view of the diagnosis, an electrocardiogram (ECG) is performed. Following the successful treatment of the pneumothorax, Helen is discharged with an outpatient appointment for medical genetics for assessment and counselling. She is referred for an MRI study of the brain.

What is the chance of Helen's daughter having the condition?

Assuming the father does not also have tuberous sclerosis, there is a 50% chance that each offspring will carry the gene. There is variable expression, i.e. individuals with the tuberous sclerosis gene will have varying degrees of the tuberous sclerosis phenotype (i.e. clinical features). Screening investigations (renal ultrasound, brain MRI) may be offered.

Several weeks later, Helen presents to the accident and emergency department with severe left flank pain and hypotension. She denies feeling feverish. Physical examination reveals left renal angle tenderness.

What investigations would you arrange and why?

- Urine dipstick and culture – to look for haematuria or evidence of a urinary tract infection
- Blood samples:
  - full blood count – to look for signs of infection
  - urea and electrolytes – to assess renal function
- Imaging:
  - renal ultrasound – to look for renal calculi or hydronephrosis, and to look for possible complications of tuberous sclerosis (Figs 10.4 & 10.5)

What does the renal ultrasound show?

There are multiple echogenic masses within the kidney without any posterior acoustic shadows. These are the typical appearances of multiple angiomyolipomas,

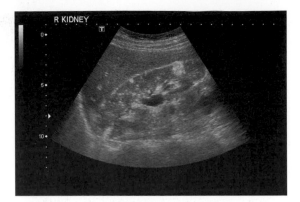

Figure 10.4 Ultrasound image of the right kidney.

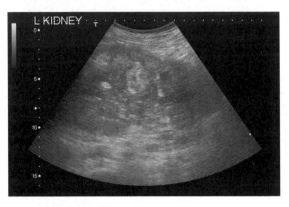

Figure 10.5 Ultrasound image of the left kidney.

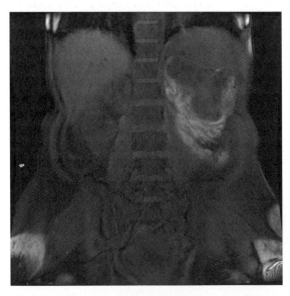

Figure 10.6 Coronal fat-suppressed T2-weighted image of the abdomen.

particularly in the context of tuberous sclerosis. Angiomyolipomas are the most common renal manifestation of tuberous sclerosis. They are benign neoplasms containing fat, smooth muscle and abnormal blood vessels. A solitary angiomyolipoma may be difficult to differentiate from a renal cell carcinoma on ultrasound imaging alone, but a CT or MRI study demonstrating fat within the mass is reassuring. Lesions without a significant fat content may require a biopsy to differentiate from a renal cell carcinoma.

What complication of tuberous sclerosis could explain her symptoms?

When small they are usually asymptomatic, but larger angiomyolipomas can cause pain and, less commonly, spontaneous haemorrhage. In this respect the ultrasound was equivocal – the margin of the left kidney appeared ill-defined, but no definite perinephric collection could be identified.

What would you do now?

Further cross-sectional imaging is necessary to further evaluate the kidneys, with either CT or MRI. In this case the patient underwent MRI (Fig. 10.6).

What does the image show?

This is a T2-weighted coronal image of the abdomen that shows an increase in signal around the left kidney. This abnormal high signal represents a perinephric collection. Given the underlying diagnosis, spontaneous haemorrhage from one of the many angiomyolipomas is the most likely cause.

How would you manage the patient now? Could further imaging be helpful?

The patient is hypotensive and has proven renal haemorrhage. She therefore requires fluid resuscitation and careful monitoring. Angiography of the renal vasculature may identify the bleeding source and enable embolization.

Helen underwent an angiogram of the left kidney to try to identify the source of the bleeding.

What do the images show?

A catheter has been positioned in the left renal artery and contrast medium has been injected. This demonstrates abnormal blood vessels in the interpolar region (Fig. 10.7, arrow) with extravasation of contrast medium

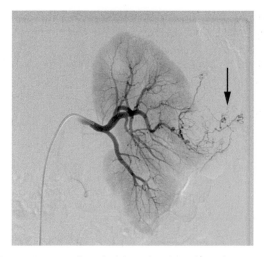

Figure 10.7 Image from the left renal angiography study.

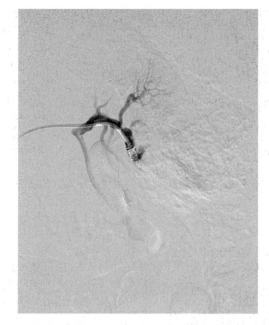

Figure 10.9 Image from the left renal angiography study.

outside the kidney (Fig. 10.8, arrow) indicating that there is active bleeding. The catheter was advanced in to a more peripheral feeding artery and the artery was then embolized. Embolization (occlusion) of a bleeding vessel may be achieved using metal coils, particulate material or tissue glue. Following embolization, no further extravasation of contrast medium was seen (Fig. 10.9), obviating the need for surgical intervention.

Helen made an uneventful recovery and was discharged home.

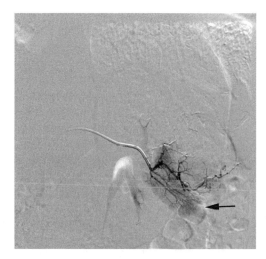

Figure 10.8 Image from the left renal angiography study.

CASE REVIEW

A 31-year-old woman presented with acute onset shortness of breath. A chest X-ray demonstrated a pneumothorax with underlying lung disease. The pneumothorax was aspirated in accordance with the BTS guidelines. An HRCT examination demonstrated multiple thin-walled cysts throughout both lungs. These radiological findings, coupled with the characteristic skin lesions (facial angiofibromas), enabled the diagnosis of tuberous sclerosis.

The patient later presents with flank pain, hypotension and haematuria. A renal ultrasound shows multiple angiomyolipomas, a common finding in tuberous sclerosis. An MRI examination demonstrates a perinephric haematoma. The patient was managed radiologically with arterial embolization and made a good recovery.

KEY POINTS

- The initial assessment of a breathless patient should be in the order: Airway, Breathing, Circulation
- Tension pneumothorax is a diagnosis that should be made clinically and treated prior to chest X-ray
- Not all spontaneous pneumothoraces require a chest drain; many can be treated with aspiration according to the BTS guidelines
- HRCT is used to assess lung parenchymal abnormalities
- Tuberous sclerosis is a relatively common multisystem disorder which is brought about by one of two genetic mutations

- Clinical features are variably expressed, and as such can present at any age from the antenatal period through to adulthood
- The condition is characterized by multiple hamartomas and tumours, most commonly the brain, skin and kidneys
- Over 50% of patients with tuberous sclerosis will have a normal IQ
- Interventional radiology techniques may be used to identify and treat acute haemorrhage, obviating the need for open surgery

Reference

Henry M, Arnold T, Harvey J. (2003) BTS guidelines for the management of spontaneous pneumothorax. *Thorax* **58** (Suppl 2), 39–52.

Case 11 A 30-year-old man with night sweats

Michael Elgood, a 30-year-old man, presents to his GP with a 2-week history of night sweats. He has recently returned from visiting his family in Jamaica (where he was born). He has no other symptoms to speak of and has no significant past medical or family history. On examination the GP identifies an enlarged lymph node in the cervical region which she estimates to be approximately 2 cm in diameter.

What are the possible causes of an enlarged lymph node?

The causes may be:
- Reactive:
  ○ tonsilitis, abscess, etc.
- Infective:
  ○ viral – Epstein–Barr virus (EBV), cytomegalovirus (CMV), HIV, rubella, measles
  ○ bacterial infection (including tuberculosis)
  ○ parasitic (e.g. toxoplasmosis)
- Neoplastic:
  ○ primary – lymphoma, acute lymphoblastic leukaemia (ALL), chronic lymphocytic leukaemia (CLL)
  ○ secondary – metastases via lymphatic spread
- Inflammatory:
  ○ sarcoid
  ○ connective tissue disease – systemic lupus erythematosus (SLE), rheumatoid arthritis
  ○ histiocytosis

Malignancies usually metastasize to local lymph nodes first – the site of the lymph node will therefore determine the most likely primary. In this case, squamous cell carcinoma of the head and neck, or a thyroid cancer would be the most likely primary malignancy to metastasize to the cervical chain.

Radiology: Clinical Cases Uncovered. By A. S. Shaw, E. M. Godfrey, A. Singh and T. F. Massoud. Published 2009 by Blackwell Publishing. ISBN 978-1-4051-8474-8.

What would you do if you were the GP?

Management of an enlarged cervical lymph node is difficult – there are a wide variety of causes, varying from benign to malignant. Neither is it an uncommon presentation – referral to hospital of every case would not be feasible.

The choice of investigation hinges on the history and examination; a 16-year-old with a sore throat should be managed differently from a 60-year-old with visible squamous cell carcinoma on the scalp. Although malignancy is less likely in younger patients, all should have their scalp, mouth, throat, ears and thyroid examined for a possible primary lesion. The axillae and groins should be examined for other enlarged lymph nodes. The spleen should be examined (because it is part of the reticuloendothelial system, it can be considered as a big lymph node).

The investigations to be considered are:
- Blood tests:
  ○ full blood count (FBC)
  ○ erythrocyte sedimentation rate (ESR)
  ○ liver function tests (LFTs)
  ○ C-reactive protein (CRP)
  ○ Paul–Bunnell test (for EBV)
  ○ HIV test
  ○ blood cultures
- Radiology:
  ○ chest X-ray
  ○ CT
- Histology:
  ○ core biopsy
  ○ excision biopsy
- Others:
  ○ Mantoux test

The history of night sweats is a concerning symptom – this should prompt earlier referral in the context of an enlarged cervical lymph node.

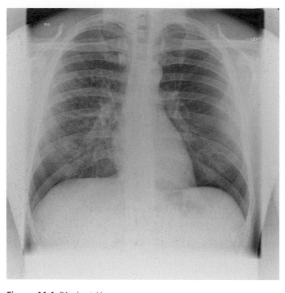

Figure 11.1 PA chest X-ray.

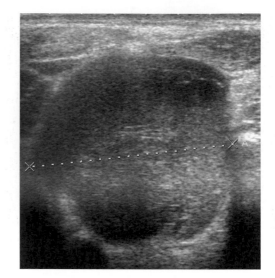

Figure 11.2 Ultrasound of the cervical node.

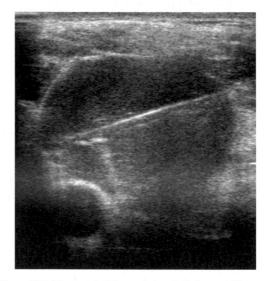

Figure 11.3 Ultrasound of the cervical node during core biopsy.

After thoroughly examining the patient (and finding nothing of note), the GP sent blood for FBC, urea and electrolytes (U+E), CRP, LFTs and the Paul–Bunnell test and HIV test (after counselling the patient appropriately). He also arranged a chest X-ray (Fig. 11.1).

He arranged to see Michael later in the week for follow-up and also to give him the results of the tests. On his return, Michael was still feeling unwell. The cervical lymph node had not changed in size. All the blood tests were normal.

What does the image show?

The lungs are clear. There is no pleural effusion. The mediastinal contour is normal. No enlarged lymph nodes are visible (the hila are normal in size, and there are no abnormal bulges from the mediastinum).

What would you do next?

Unfortunately, a normal chest X-ray and blood tests, while reassuring to an extent, do not exclude the possibility that there is an underlying malignancy involving Michael's cervical lymph node. Because no clear cause has been identified, it would be sensible to continue investigating him. A reasonable next step would be to request an ultrasound-guided biopsy of the lymph node. NB Some practitioners would advocate lymph node excision rather than core biopsy.

I *The GP requests an urgent lymph node biopsy.*

What do the images show?

Figure 11.2 shows a 3-cm rounded hypoechoic structure. This would be consistent with an abnormal enlarged lymph node. Figure 11.3 shows the same lymph node being biopsied with a needle running through it.

The biopsy samples were sent to histology. Michael returned to the GP for the results, which showed granulomas within reactive lymphoid tissue.

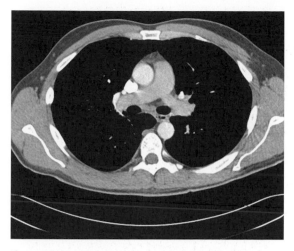

Figure 11.4 Axial CT of the thorax at the level of the hila.

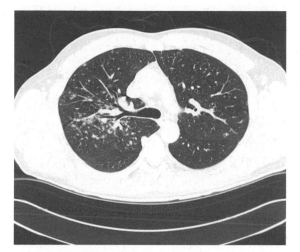

Figure 11.5 Axial CT of the thorax.

What does the presence of granulomas suggest?

A granuloma is a nodule of epithelioid macrophages, often surrounded by a ring of lymphocytes. They are the hallmark of granulomatous diseases, which include tuberculosis, sarcoidosis, Crohn's disease and Wegener's granulomatosis. Granulomas in tuberculosis tend to be caseating (i.e. the centre is filled with necrotic tissue); however, on small samples of tissue this can be difficult to establish.

The presence of granulomas in the biopsy tissue narrows the differential considerably; tuberculosis and sarcoid are now the most likely candidates. Both would be consistent with a history of night sweats.

What would you do next?

A Mantoux test would be advised to investigate for tuberculosis. A chest CT would be useful, because both tuberculosis and sarcoidosis often affect the lung parenchyma and the thoracic lymph nodes.

I *A Mantoux test was performed, which was negative.*

What do the images show?

Figure 11.4 shows the hila on CT. This confirms that there are no enlarged hilar lymph nodes (as noted on the previous chest X-ray). Figure 11.5 is an HRCT image showing perilymphatic nodules. Figure 11.6 is a sagittal reformatted image that demonstrates the predilection the nodules have for the oblique fissure. This is known as

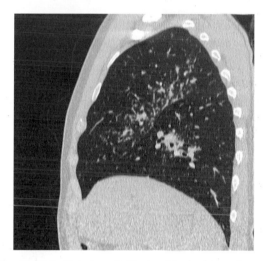

Figure 11.6 Sagittal reformatted image of the lung parenchyma.

fissural beading and is a sign strongly suggestive of sarcoidosis.

The CT report described the features and favoured sarcoidosis as the most likely diagnosis. Box 11.1 gives an outline of sarcoidosis and Box 11.2 describes the staging of sarcoidosis according to the chest X-ray.

Following the CT examination, Michael was referred to a respiratory physician. After explaining the diagnosis, the physician prescribed a short course of steroids which improved his symptoms. He was followed up at 6 months.

At follow-up Michael complained of fatigue and breathlessness. His full blood count results are given in Box 11.3.

Box 11.1 Sarcoidosis

- Sarcoidosis is a chronic non-caseating granulomatous disease of unknown aetiology
- It is a multisystem disorder that most frequently affects the lungs
- It is more common in the West and particularly in people of West African descent
- Women are more commonly affected than men
- The disease usually presents in early adulthood

Box 11.2 Stages of sarcoidosis

Stage 0	Normal
Stage I	Bilateral hilar adenopathy
Stage II	Bilateral hilar adenopathy and reticular opacities
Stage III	Reticular opacities alone
Stage IV	Fibrosis (honeycombing), with parenchymal distortion

Box 11.3 Full blood count at follow-up

Hb 7.5 g/dL (normal range 13–17)
Mean cell volume (MCV) 85 fl (80–100)
Platelets 60 × 10^9/l (150–400)
White cell count (WCC) 3.2 × 10^9/L (4–11)
Neutrophils 1.2 × 10^9/L (4–11)

Box 11.4 Features of sarcoidosis

- General:
  - fever/night sweats
  - weight loss
  - hypercalcaemia
- Pulmonary:
  - pulmonary fibrosis
- Lymphatic:
  - lymph node enlargement – typically hilar but can be anywhere
  - splenomegaly
- Dermatological:
  - erythema nodosum
  - lupus pernio
- Cardiac:
  - cor pulmonale (right ventricular failure secondary to pulmonary fibrosis)
  - heart block
  - arrhythmias
- Ocular:
  - uveitis
  - retinal vasculitis
  - keratoconjunctivitis
- Neurologic:
  - mononeuritis multiplex
  - septic meningitis
  - seizures
  - vasculitis
  - stroke or transient ischaemic attack

What do the blood results show?

There is a normocytic anaemia. The white cells and platelets are also low. This would be classed as a pancytopenia.

The respiratory physician requests an ultrasound of the abdomen (Fig. 11.7).

What does the image show?

This is an ultrasound image of the spleen showing that it measures 16.5 cm. It appears heterogeneous. Both these features are abnormal (the spleen is normally <13 cm in maximal diameter).

Is this a feature of sarcoidosis?

Yes – splenomegaly can occur in a wide variety of conditions. Sarcoidosis is one of them. Box 11.4 lists the various features of sarcoidosis. Box 11.5 lists the possible causes of splenomegaly.

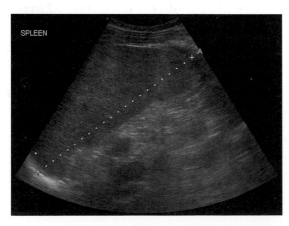

SPLEEN

Figure 11.7 Ultrasound of the left upper quadrant.

Box 11.5 Causes of splenomegaly

- Infective:
  - ○ bacterial, e.g. Osler's subacute bacterial endocarditis
  - ○ viral, e.g. CMV, EBV, HIV
  - ○ protozoal, e.g. malaria
- Lymphoproliferative:
  - ○ lymphoma
- Myeloproliferative:
  - ○ polycythaemia
  - ○ essential thrombocythaemia
  - ○ myelofibrosis
  - ○ leukaemia
- Congestive:
  - ○ congestive heart disease
  - ○ portal hypertension
- Inflammatory:
  - ○ Felty's syndrome
  - ○ sarcoidosis
- Haemolytic anaemias:
  - ○ autoimmune haemolytic anaemia
- Storage/deposition disorders:
  - ○ Gaucher's disease
  - ○ amyloidosis

What is the link between splenomegaly and the blood results?

An enlarged spleen, whatever the underlying cause, may give rise to hypersplenism. This is a condition characterized by splenomegaly, pancytopenia, normal or hyperplastic bone marrow and response to splenectomy.

Michael was referred to a haematologist who performed a bone marrow biopsy. The bone marrow biopsy was normal. The haematologist therefore discussed the option of splenectomy which Michael agreed to undergo.

Are there any precautions that are necessary prior to elective splenectomy?

The spleen's major immune function is against encapsulated bacteria. These include *Streptococcus pneumoniae*, *Neisseria meningitidis* and *Haemophilis influenzae*. It is therefore standard practice to immunize against these organisms prior to elective splenectomy. The patient should be counselled that they are at increased risk of malaria. Many centres also prescribe life-long antibiotic prophylaxis for those undergoing splenectomy.

Michael underwent a laparoscopic splenectomy. His pancytopenia subsequently resolved. He remained under the care of the respiratory team for monitoring of his sarcoid.

CASE REVIEW

A 30-year-old man presents to his GP with a history of nights sweats. The GP finds an enlarged cervical lymph node. On examination there is no obvious underlying cause. Routine blood tests and a plain chest X-ray are normal.

The GP arranges a lymph node biopsy which shows granulomas. A Mantoux test for tuberculosis is negative. A chest CT examination identifies perilymphatic nodules and beading of the oblique fissure, consistent with sarcoidosis.

The patient is treated with a course of oral steroids and makes a clinical recovery.

Six months later, the patient is reviewed and complains of lethargy and shortness of breath. A full blood count reveals pancytopenia. An ultrasound examination identifies splenomegaly.

The patient is referred for laparoscopic splenectomy after the appropriate vaccinations have been given. He makes a good recovery and his full blood count improves.

KEY POINTS

- An enlarged cervical lymph node is a concerning sign that should be evaluated carefully
- If an enlarged cervical lymph node is found, the scalp, mouth, throat, ears and thyroid should be examined for a possible primary malignancy
- A wide variety of conditions can cause enlargement of cervical lymph nodes. Some of these may be diagnosed via a blood test, e.g. glandular fever/infectious mononucleosis
- In cases where no cause is identified, an ultrasound-guided core biopsy of an enlarged cervical lymph node is a reasonable strategy
- Granulomas are characteristic of a relatively small number of conditions
- Not all patients with sarcoidosis have bi-hilar lymphadenopathy, although this is a common feature seen on a chest X-ray
- Sarcoidosis is a relatively common granulomatous disease of unknown aetiology. It most often affects the lungs
- CT findings in sarcoidosis include lymph node enlargement, perilymphatic nodules and fissural beading
- Many different conditions can cause splenomegaly
- Splenomegaly of any cause can give rise to hypersplenism, a cause of pancytopenia
- Splenectomy is the treatment of choice for hypersplenism
- Vaccines against *Streptococcus pneumoniae*, *Haemophilus influenzae* and *Neisseria meningitides* should be given prior to splenectomy

Case 12 A 27-year-old woman involved in a road traffic accident

A 27-year-old law student, Amanda Smith, is brought to the local hospital by paramedics after they were called to the scene of a major road traffic accident. The history from the paramedic team is that Amanda had been the driver of a car that had been travelling at approximately 50 mph (80 kph) in heavy rain when she had lost control. Witnesses to the accident said that the car had left the road and rolled twice before coming to a standstill. Passing motorists immediately called the emergency services which were quickly in attendance. Amanda was conscious on arrival of the emergency services but all three occupants of the car needed to be cut from the wreckage by the fire brigade. Amanda's friends had not yet been freed from the car.

On arrival in to the resuscitation area of the accident and emergency department what should be the immediate management steps?

The 'ABC' protocol should be followed, in particular the Advanced Trauma Life Support (ATLS) guidelines as set out by the American College of Surgeons Committee on Trauma. A brief overview of the key points is given in Box 12.1. Many of the initial stages will have been carried out en route to the hospital by the paramedic team as a matter of course.

Initial assessment:
- Airway and cervical spine – Amanda's cervical spine has been immobilized in a hard collar. Her airway is patent; she is able to converse with the doctors and is not complaining of any pain in her neck. She is continued on 100% oxygen via a tight-fitting face mask.
- Breathing – Her blood oxygen saturation is 98% and her breath sounds are normal with good bilateral air entry. No thoracic injuries apparent.

Radiology: Clinical Cases Uncovered. By A. S. Shaw, E. M. Godfrey, A. Singh and T. F. Massoud. Published 2009 by Blackwell Publishing. ISBN 978-1-4051-8474-8.

- Circulation – Amanda has a pulse rate of 104 beats/minute, blood pressure of 98/59 mmHg. Her peripheries are cold and she looks pale with a capillary refill time of 3 seconds. She has only one peripheral intravenous line so another large-bore cannula is sited in the other arm. Intravenous fluids are commenced. Blood samples are sent to the laboratory for assessment and cross-matching.
- Disability – Her Glasgow Coma Score (GCS) is 15, pupils are normal size, bilaterally equal and reactive to light.
- Exposure – She is found to have some bruising in her right upper quadrant and right loin area and is complaining of severe pain in this region. Amanda has no pain in her pelvis and no injuries are identified in the perineal and genital regions. A digital rectal examination and assessment of anal tone is normal. No other obvious injury is identified after a brief assessment of her neurological and musculoskeletal systems.

What should you do next?

At present Amanda is tachycardic and hypotensive, which is of great concern in a young patient. Younger patients tend to be able to compensate following blood loss better than older patients. In view of this, it was decided to fluid resuscitate Amanda in the first instance and obtain imaging within the emergency department. A trauma series is requested by the physician.

What are the standard trauma series plain X-rays that should be obtained?

The imaging protocols for major trauma vary between different centres and will depend upon the facilities and personnel available. As an absolute bare minimum, the trauma series should include:
- Lateral X-ray of the cervical spine
- Frontal chest X-ray
- AP view of the pelvis
- Further imaging (plain films, ultrasound or CT) as clinically indicated

> **Box 12.1 Brief outline of the Advanced Trauma Life Support guidelines as set out by the American College of Surgeons Committee on Trauma**
>
> **Primary survey**
>
> **A Airway and cervical spine**
> - Secure a definitive airway
> - Concurrent and immediate stabilization of the cervical spine
> - Assume a cervical spine injury in any patient with trauma
>
> **B Breathing**
> - Adequate oxygenation and ventilation
> - Expose chest and examine
> - Treat life-threatening chest injuries immediately
>
> **C Circulation**
> - Assess level of consciousness and cardiovascular system
> - Immediate identification and control of external bleeding initially by direct manual pressure on the wound
> - Fluid resuscitation as necessary
>
> **D Disability**
> - Pupillary size and reaction
> - Glasgow Coma Score
>
> **E Exposure and environmental control**
> - Completely undress the patient to assess the whole body from head to toe including every orifice using a 'log roll'
> - Cover the patient with warm blankets or external warming device after completing the assessment
>
> **Secondary survey**
> Begin only when the primary survey is complete, resuscitation and management steps are underway and the patient is beginning to stabilize
> - Full history
> - Careful examination from head to toe
> - Further imaging as required

However, many major trauma centres have now abandoned some or all of this in favour of a CT of the whole body for those patients who are sufficiently stable. The rationale for this is that the whole procedure can be performed quickly, gives an unparalleled view of all regions, and it is both more sensitive and specific in diagnosing injuries than any other imaging modality in this setting. The only disadvantage is the radiation dose, but this is far outweighed by the risk of missing a major injury.

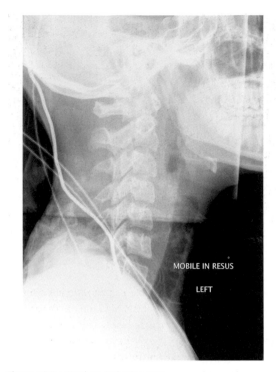

Figure 12.1 Lateral cervical spine X-ray.

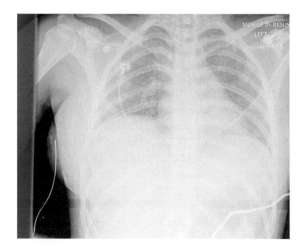

Figure 12.2 Frontal chest X-ray.

Is this cervical spine image a satisfactory X-ray? Do you see any abnormality?

A lateral view of the cervical spine should include the skull base superiorly and the T1 vertebra inferiorly. On this image (Fig. 12.1), the C7 vertebra is only partially visible and the T1 vertebra is not visible. Evaluation of the cervical spine needs to be careful and methodical.

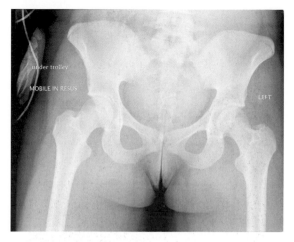

Figure 12.3 AP view of the pelvis.

> **Box 12.2 FAST scan**
>
> Ultrasound is used to look for the presence of fluid in four places:
>
> **1** Pericardium
> **2** Perihepatic
> **3** Perisplenic
> **4** Pelvis
>
>   The presence of free fluid in patients who are unstable from a cardiovascular perspective is an indication for laparotomy. The procedure may be carried out in a few minutes and has a high sensitivity and specificity in experienced hands. It should not be used for assessing the retroperitoneal space, the solid organs, bowel or vascular injuries

Alignment of the vertebral bodies and skull base should be checked along the anterior and posterior borders of the vertebral bodies, together with the posterior elements. The pre-vertebral soft tissues should be assessed for swelling (to indicate haemorrhage) if the patient has not been intubated. Even when the imaging (any imaging) is normal, it is crucial to remember that 'clearing' a cervical spine is a clinical decision that can only really be made following examination on a conscious and responsive patient. In this case, no abnormality can be seen in the upper cervical spine.

If facing difficulties imaging the lower cervical and upper thoracic vertebra, what other strategies can be employed?

• Traction may be applied to the patient's shoulders by two assistants while taking the lateral X-ray
• A 'swimmers' view of the lower cervical and upper thoracic vertebrae can be obtained
• If there is any doubt or clinical concern then a CT examination of the cervical spine should be performed

A repeat X-ray was requested to obtain better views of the C7 vertebral body and is found to be normal as are the chest and pelvis X-rays (Figs 12.2 & 12.3). The clinicians remain concerned about Amanda's clinical state and are unwilling to transfer her to the radiology department for a CT.

What other options are available for imaging the abdomen?

Ultrasound, or more specifically, focused assessment with sonography for trauma – a FAST scan (Box 12.2) – may be used in this situation. This looks for the presence of fluid in the pericardium and peritoneal spaces and may help decision-making in the trauma setting. However, in order to gain the most benefit it is vital that one understands its shortcomings. Ultrasound does not enable reliable evaluation of the solid organs for traumatic injuries, it is of limited value in the retroperitoneal space and has no role in the evaluation of mesenteric or bowel injury.

As part of the imaging assessment, Amanda undergoes a FAST scan which demonstrates free fluid within her abdomen. She begins to complain of worsening severe abdominal pain and appears drowsy and confused. Pale, cold and 'clammy', Amanda's pulse is 120 beats/minute and her blood pressure is 80/50 mmHg.

What is the diagnosis?

Amanda has haemorrhagic shock. The clinical features of tachycardia and hypotension unresponsive to fluid resuscitation, together with abdominal bruising and pain, and a positive diagnosis of haemoperitoneum on the FAST scan indicate that there is active intra-abdominal haemorrhage.

What should be your next investigation?

No further radiological investigations should be performed at this stage. The patient is unstable from a cardiovascular perspective and any further delay may be potentially fatal. In this circumstance, the patient should be transferred to the operating theatre for a laparotomy.

Amanda was transferred to the operating theatre. At laparotomy, the surgical team finds a large amount of blood within the peritoneal cavity originating from a complex laceration of the right lobe of the liver. Despite their best efforts, they are unable to control the bleeding and are compelled to perform a partial hepatectomy. Following surgery, Amanda was transferred to the intensive therapy unit (ITU).

There is still a very important step that needs to be carried out before her initial trauma assessment can be completed following her accident, what is it?

The secondary survey (Box 12.1). Now that Amanda has returned from theatre and her immediate life-threatening injury has been addressed, it would be a good opportunity to carry out a secondary survey and look carefully for any other injuries that were missed in the primary survey.

Other than bruising over her right elbow, no other injuries are identified. X-rays are taken of Amanda's right elbow.

What do these images show?

There is elevation of the anterior fat pad (which lies just anterior to the distal humerus) implying a joint effusion (Fig. 12.4, upper arrow). There is a fracture seen through the head of the radius (Fig. 12.4, lower arrow).

The elbow is immobilized in plaster. Unfortunately, Amanda's condition fails to improve over the next 48 hours and she continues to require intensive support. A chest X-ray is taken (Fig. 12.5).

What does this image show?

The film has been taken AP in a semi-erect position. There is an endotracheal tube *in situ*. There is a right internal jugular venous line with its tip in the superior vena cava. There is an intercostal chest drain *in situ* at the right lung base with a moderate volume right-sided pleural effusion (note that the costophrenic recess is obscured). The lungs are otherwise clear and the heart appears normal. Below the diaphragm, the high density material represents surgical packing from the recent hepatectomy.

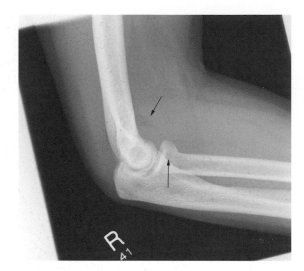

Figure 12.4 Lateral view of the right elbow.

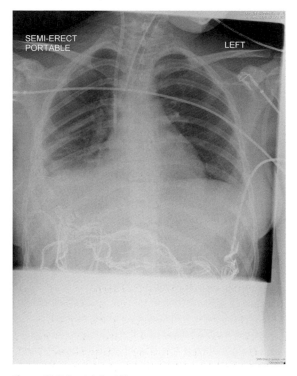

Figure 12.5 Frontal chest X-ray.

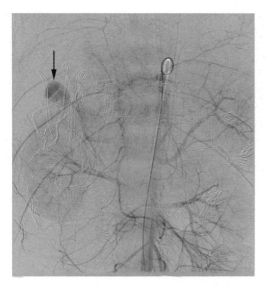

Figure 12.6 Digital subtraction angiogram performed with a pigtail catheter in the aorta.

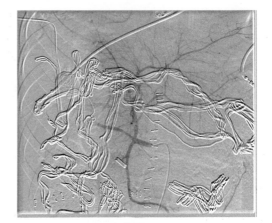

Figure 12.7 Digital subtraction angiogram performed with a pigtail catheter in the aorta following embolization.

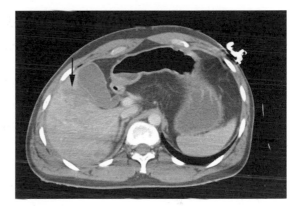

Figure 12.8 Contrast enhanced axial CT image through the abdomen.

What is the most likely cause of Amanda's persistent haemodynamic instability?

There may be a source of continued bleeding that was either not identified or that has developed since surgery.

How might you investigate this?

Angiography of the liver may be invaluable in this situation. It would provide a minimally invasive way of identifying any occult source of bleeding as well as having the potential to stop the bleeding by embolization.

Amanda is taken to the angiography suite where the interventional radiologist performs an angiogram of the liver via a catheter inserted in to the right superficial femoral artery.

What do these images show?

There are artefacts from the surgical packs. However, in Fig. 12.6 (arrow), a 3.5-cm diameter opacity is seen arising from the hepatic artery. This is a large pseudoaneurysm, presumably related to surgery, which is at high risk of rupture. Following the placement of several metal coils within the aneurysm and a smaller coil placed in the feeding branch of the right hepatic artery, stasis of blood flow is now seen with no filling of the aneurysm (Fig. 12.7).

Following the procedure, Amanda returns to the ITU and her condition soon begins to stabilize. She subsequently makes an uneventful recovery.

Amanda's friend Adam was sitting in the rear seat behind her and was also injured in the accident; he was not wearing a seat belt. He complains of upper abdominal pain. Other than bruising over the right side of the abdomen, Adam's primary and secondary survey reveal no other obvious injuries. He was referred for a CT examination of the abdomen and pelvis.

What do these images show?

There is a liver laceration extending in to the gallbladder fossa (Fig. 12.8, arrow) with a pocket of blood just deep to the inferior edge of the liver (Fig. 12.9, arrow).

Box 12.3 American Association for the Surgery of Trauma grading of liver trauma

- *Grade 1* – A subcapsular haematoma measuring <1 cm deep, a capsular avulsion, a superficial parenchymal laceration <1 cm deep, or isolated periportal blood tracking
- *Grade 2* – A parenchymal laceration 1–3 cm deep or a parenchymal and/or subcapsular haematoma 1–3 cm thick
- *Grade 3* – A parenchymal laceration >3 cm deep or a parenchymal and/or subcapsular haematoma >3 cm in diameter
- *Grade 4* – A parenchymal and/or subcapsular haematoma >10 cm in diameter, lobar destruction or devascularization
- *Grade 5* – Global destruction or devascularization of the liver
- *Grade 6* – Hepatic avulsion

Having both been on the same side of the car and exposed to similar forces, it is perhaps unsurprising that Amanda and Adam have similar injuries. However, Adam has a much lower grade injury and is haemodynamically stable; he was managed conservatively.

How is liver trauma categorized?

The American Association for the Surgery of Trauma (AAST) defines a six-point scale of liver trauma, summarized in Box 12.3.

John, the third passenger, was sitting in the front passenger seat and was also injured in the accident. The paramedic crew informed the emergency department that he had been found unconscious but had been wearing a seat belt. He awoke in the ambulance and remembers nothing of the accident. John complains of severe pain along the back of his neck and says that he cannot feel his legs. Following the primary survey John is found to have marked cervical spine tenderness, in particular at the level of C5 and C6. There is also extensive bruising across the right side of his chest and root of the neck. Examination of the chest reveals reduced air entry and hyper-resonance on percussion on the right side. From a cardiovascular perspective, he is stable. X-rays are taken of the cervical spine, chest and pelvis.

How would you interpret this image?

This X-ray (Fig. 12.10) is not adequate as the C5 vertebra is the lowest vertebral body imaged. The artefact that can

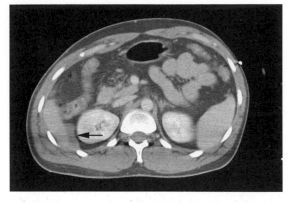

Figure 12.9 Contrast enhanced axial CT image through the abdomen.

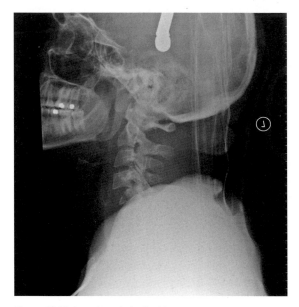

Figure 12.10 Lateral cervical spine X-ray.

be seen is from the cervical spine collar immobilizing the neck. As one follows the line down the anterior border of the vertebral bodies, there is a clear step posteriorly at the level of the C5 vertebral body. The same is noted following the alignment of the posterior border of the vertebral bodies. The posterior elements cannot be clearly seen. There is also an oblique fracture of the C5 vertebral body. The pattern of the injury is typical of a hyperflexion injury. Given the degree of posterior displacement of the C5 vertebral body, some degree of compression of the spinal cord seems inevitable.

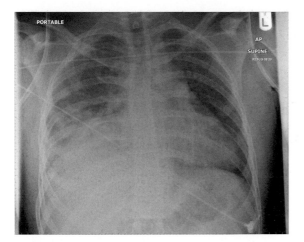

Figure 12.11 Frontal chest X-ray.

PART 2: CASES

> **Box 12.4 Major trauma CT protocol**
>
> - Unenhanced images (to identify blood):
>   - head
>   - cervical spine
>   - thorax
>   - abdomen
>   - pelvis
> - Arterial phase images (to look for an arterial injury):
>   - thorax
>   - abdomen
> - Portal venous phase images (to assess the abdominal viscera):
>   - abdomen
>   - pelvis
> - Delayed images (if there is suspected ureteric or bladder injury):
>   - abdomen
>   - pelvis

How would you interpret this image?

Importantly, the film has been taken with the patient supine (Fig. 12.11). There is consolidation and pleural fluid in the right hemithorax. In addition, there are fractures of the right second and seventh ribs. Given the clinical context, it is almost certain that these findings represent pulmonary contusions and a haemothorax. Furthermore, clinical examination suggested a pneumothorax on the right. This has not been excluded by this image; it has been taken with the patient supine.

The pelvic X-ray is normal but further assessment in the primary survey reveals sensory loss below the level of T4, hyper-reflxia and absent anal tone. A right-sided intercostal chest drain was inserted.

What would you do now?

As a result of the initial investigations we know that John has:
- Undergone major trauma to his head, neck and chest at least
- Suffered a period of amnesia
- A major cervical spine injury with cord compromise
- A right-sided thoracic injury

An urgent CT examination is required to fully assess his injuries. The imaging protocol for major trauma such as this should include from head to pelvis, irrespective of what is or is not suspected. The extra time taken to acquire the images is a matter of seconds. The risk from the additional radiation is negligible when compared with the risk of not identifying an occult injury. A typical protocol is given in Box 12.4.

What do the images in Figs 12.12–12.16 demonstrate?

There is a fracture of C1 with disruption of the bony ring. There are complex comminuted fractures of the C5 and C6 vertebral bodies with posterior displacement of the C5 vertebral body posteriorly in to the spinal canal.

What abnormalities can you see on John's chest CT?

There is a right-sided haemopneumothorax with extensive right-sided pulmonary contusions. An intercostal drain is seen in a satisfactory position posteriorly. There is also a fracture through the sternum with a retrosternal haematoma lying in front of the ascending aorta (Figs 12.17 & 12.18).

What does a sternal fracture signify?

Fractures of the sternum indicate severe forces involved in the mechanism of injury. A similar conclusion can be drawn from injuries to the first and second ribs.

What further imaging required?

John requires an urgent MRI study of his spine to assess the level of injury sustained to his spinal cord and the other soft tissues of the neck.

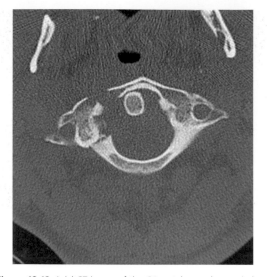

Figure 12.12 Axial CT image of the C1 vertebra on bone window.

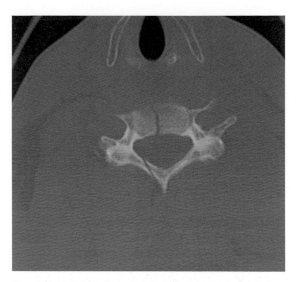

Figure 12.14 Axial CT image of the C6 vertebra on bone window.

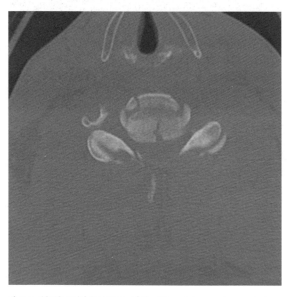

Figure 12.13 Axial CT image of the C5 vertebra on bone window.

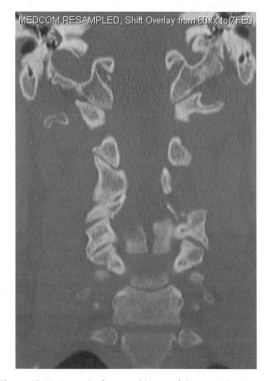

Figure 12.15 Coronal reformatted image of the cervical spine on bone window.

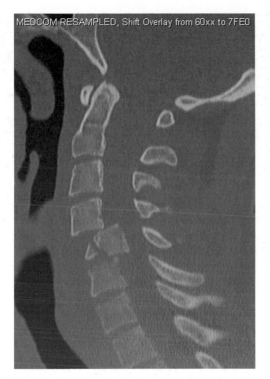

Figure 12.16 Sagittal reformatted image of the cervical spine on bone window.

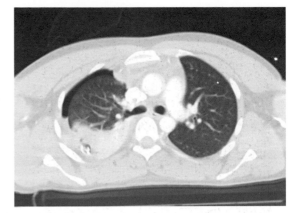

Figure 12.18 Axial contrast enhanced CT image of the thorax on lung windows.

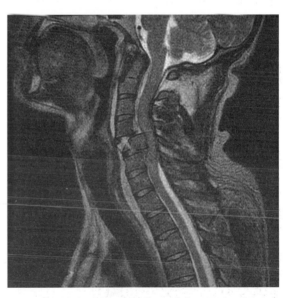

Figure 12.19 Sagittal T2-weighted MRI of the cervical and upper thoracic spine.

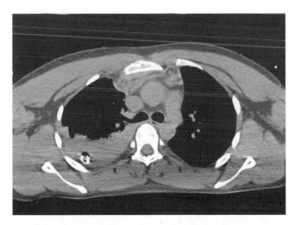

Figure 12.17 Axial unenhanced CT image of the thorax on soft tissue windows.

What does this study demonstrate?

There is significant retropulsion of the unstable fractured C5 vertebral body which is encroaching upon the spinal cord (Fig. 12.19). The spinal cord itself demonstrates a slight increase in signal, signifying cord oedema secondary to compression, but is intact.

How would this be managed?

John requires urgent neurosurgical decompression of the cord and fixation of the cervical spine fractures.

He was taken immediately to theatre for surgery and made a full recovery with no permanent neurological deficit.

CASE REVIEW

Amanda Smith and two of her friends were involved in a high speed road traffic accident which required them to be cut free from the wreckage of the car. On arrival at hospital, Amanda was managed according to ATLS guidelines but was cardiovascularly unstable. Plain films excluded thoracic haemorrhage and a FAST scan identified peritoneal haemorrhage. In haemorrhagic shock, Amanda was taken to theatre for a laparotomy where a severe liver injury was treated with a right hepatectomy. Amanda remained unstable and a few days later, a pseudoaneurysm of the hepatic artery was identified and embolized.

Amanda's friend Adam had been unrestrained in a rear passenger seat at the time of the collision. On arrival in hospital he had evidence of right-sided abdominal injuries. A CT study identified a laceration of the right liver. He was managed conservatively and made an uneventful recovery.

A second friend, John, had been in the front passenger seat. He arrived in hospital with head, neck and thoracic injuries apparent, but was stable from a cardiovascular perspective. In accordance with ATLS guidelines, a chest drain was inserted and he underwent a CT study from head to pelvis. The CT confirmed cervical spine fractures with a large retropulsed fragment at C5. There was a right-sided haemopneumothorax and pulmonary contusions. An MRI study confirmed oedema of the cord and surgical fixation of the cervical spine was undertaken without delay. John made a full recovery.

KEY POINTS

- Patients in high speed accidents often sustain injuries to more than one body part
- A precise efficient assessment is vital to optimize survival and reduce morbidity
- Management according to ATLS guidelines is crucial
- Imaging should be used to facilitate patient management
- Unstable patients should not have a diagnostic laparotomy delayed by imaging
- Plain films, ultrasound, CT, MRI and interventional radiology all have a role
- Ultrasound may be used to look for fluid (FAST scan)
- Ultrasound should *not* be used to look for solid organ injuries
- CT is the gold standard imaging survey in the acute situation
- The risk of missing an injury far outweighs the risk of radiation in polytrauma

A 30-year-old man with painful swollen fingers

David Smiles, a 30-year-old man presents to his GP with painful swollen fingers. They have been getting progressively worse over the previous 2 weeks. His toes are also swollen and tender. He feels otherwise well. He has psoriasis, as do several members of his mother's family, but has no other medical conditions.

What is psoriasis?

Psoriasis is a skin condition with a variety of different manifestations. The most common form (plaque psoriasis) presents as raised 'plaques', covered with silver scaly skin.

The aetiology of psoriasis has a strong genetic component. Environmental factors (such as stress, smoking, drugs) are thought to be involved in triggering and exacerbating the disease. Box 13.1 gives some important signs to look for on examination of skin lesions.

On examination there are psoriatic plaques at both elbows. There is pitting and onycholysis of the nails. There is a symmetrical non-deforming polyarthropathy affecting the fingers and toes with soft tissue swelling. The metacarpophalangeal, metatarsophalangeal and interphalangeal joints are tender and boggy on palpation, suggesting that there is active synovitis.

What is the differential diagnosis here?

Although the history of psoriasis is a helpful clue, it is important to remember that there are other possible causes of this patient's symptoms. In general, the differential diagnosis for a symmetrical polyarthropathy is predominantly:
- Rheumatoid arthritis
- Seronegative arthritis (including psoriatic arthritis)
- Viral, e.g. after parvovirus B19

Radiology: Clinical Cases Uncovered. By A. S. Shaw, E. M. Godfrey, A. Singh and T. F. Massoud. Published 2009 by Blackwell Publishing. ISBN 978-1-4051-8474-8.

What is the significance of the nail changes?

The nail changes in psoriasis occur much more frequently in those patients who have, or will go on to develop psoriatic arthritis.

What are the seronegative arthritides?

The seronegative arthritides (Box 13.2) are a diverse group of inflammatory joint conditions in patients with a negative rheumatoid factor. They share a number of common features:
- Increased incidence of HLA B27 (Box 13.3)
- Inflammation of tendon insertion sites (enthesitis)
- Sacroiliitis and spondylitis (inflammation of the joints of the spine)
- Extra-articular manifestations such as uveitis, aortitis and upper zone pulmonary fibrosis

What tests would you arrange at this point?

- Full blood count – the white cell count may be raised in acute inflammation
- Erythrocyte sedimentation rate – raised in systemic inflammatory disorders
- Urea and electrolytes – to look for renal involvement
- Urate – often tested when gout is suspected, although it may be normal even in acute gout
- Antinuclear antibody – positive in systemic lupus erythematosus (SLE) and some patients with rheumatoid arthritis
- Rheumatoid factor – positive in around 80% of patients with rheumatoid arthritis
- Urine dipstick – haematuria would suggest renal involvement, e.g. in SLE
- Plain X-rays of the hands and feet

Joint aspiration should be considered, particularly if septic arthritis is a possibility. In practice this is much more important in the context of an acute monoarthritis. It is rarely necessary with a symmetrical polyarthritis.

> **Box 13.1 Useful signs to look for on examination of the skin**
>
> - *Auspitz's sign.* Plaques that, when removed, reveal bleeding underlying the skin. This is typical of psoriasis
> - *Koebner reaction.* Skin lesions appear in scratches. This is typical of psoriasis
> - *Nikolsky's sign.* Superficial layer of skin slides over the underlying layer. This is not typical of psoriasis at all, and is more suggestive of pemphigus or staphylococcal scalded skin syndrome

> **Box 13.2 The seronegative arthritides**
>
> - *Psoriatic arthritis*
> - *Reactive arthritis.* This group of conditions is triggered by infection (often genitourinary or gastrointestinal). As well as arthritis, extra-articular manifestations are particularly common: uveitis, conjunctivitis, skin lesions (such as circinate balanitis or keratoderma blennorrhagica) and occasionally heart valve abnormalities such as aortic regurgitation. Reactive arthritis includes the syndrome formerly known as Reiter's syndrome. The term is not encouraged although still in use – Hans Reiter was convicted as a Nazi war criminal because of his experiments on a new typhus vaccine that killed hundreds of prisoners of war
> - *Enteropathic arthritis.* This arises as two distinct forms:
>   1 An axial arthritis (particularly affecting the sacroiliac joints and the spine) that is generally unrelated to bowel disease activity
>   2 A peripheral small joint arthritis that varies in severity with bowel disease activity
> - *Ankylosing spondylitis.* This is a disease of the spine and sacroiliac joints. Progressive inflammation can lead to joint fusion (ankylosis) in severe cases. HLA B27 is found in over 90% of cases. Classic radiological features include syndesmophytes (bony spurs that grow between adjacent vertebral bodies) which may eventually fuse to give the appearance of a 'bamboo' spine

The urine dipstick is clear. The GP arranges the above blood tests and requests plain X-rays of the hands and feet. She prescribes paracetamol and ibuprofen for analgesia, and arranges to see David later in the week with the initial results (autoantibody tests will take longer than this).

> **Box 13.3 HLA B27**
>
> HLA B27 is one of a variety of cell surface molecules that may be expressed as part of the major histocompatibility complex (MHC). Class I MHC molecules, including HLA B27, are involved in the expression of antigen to CD8 T cells. There is a wide variation between individuals as to which HLA genes they inherit. Individuals who inherit HLA B27 appear to be more susceptible to a number of diseases, in particular the seronegative arthritides. The strongest association is with ankylosing spondylitis.

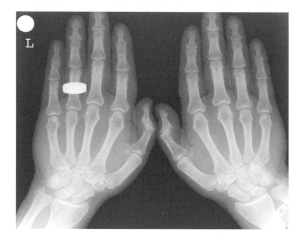

Figure 13.1 X-ray of both hands.

What do the images show?

The bones of the hands (Fig. 13.1) are unremarkable with normal joint spaces and no erosions. The fingers are 'sausage-shaped' because of swollen soft tissues. There is a destructive arthropathy predominantly affecting the distal interphalangeal (DIP) joints of the feet (Fig. 13.2), leading to loss of joint space. There is also acro-osteolysis affecting the second to fourth toes bilaterally – this is resorption of the terminal tufts of the distal phalanges. Of note, there is no periarticular osteopenia.

These features show contrasting ends of the spectrum of psoriatic arthritis. The hands are normal aside from soft tissue swelling (which is a non-specific finding and may be seen in a variety of arthritides). The feet show characteristic features of relatively advanced psoriatic arthritis: acro-osteolysis and a destructive arthropathy predominantly of the DIP joints. The absence of periarticular osteopenia is significant as this would be suggestive of rheumatoid arthritis.

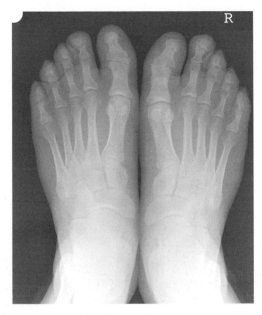

Figure 13.2 X-ray of both feet.

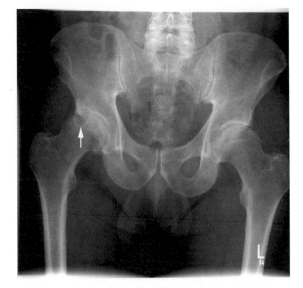

Figure 13.3 AP view of the right hip demonstrating loss of joint space, sclerosis and a subchondral cyst (arrow).

What are the different patterns of psoriatic arthritis?

Five types are recognized:

1 *Symmetrical.* This form can be clinically indistinguishable from rheumatoid arthritis, but is differentiated by the presence of psoriasis and the absence of rheumatoid factor.
2 *Asymmetrical.* This may affect one or several joints.
3 *Arthritis mutilans.* This is the most severe form, and thankfully the least common. Characteristic features include telescoping of the fingers (clinically) and 'pencil in cup' deformity (radiologically).
4 *Distal interphalangeal joint predominant.* Nail changes may be particularly prominent in this form of the disease.
5 *Spondylitis.* This occurs in 40% of patients with psoriatic arthritis, often alongside the other patterns of involvement.

Psoriasis, via increased skin cell turnover, can also predispose to gout.

What are the typical features of osteoarthritis?

There are four cardinal radiological signs of osteoarthritis (Fig. 13.3):

1 Loss of joint space
2 Subchondral sclerosis
3 Osteophytes
4 Subchondral cysts

What are the typical features of rheumatoid arthritis?

1 Loss of joint space (similar to other arthritides)
2 Juxta-articular osteopenia
3 Soft tissue swelling
4 Marginal erosions
5 Deformity tends to be greater than in other arthritides (aside from arthritis mutilans)
These are shown in Figures 13.4–13.6.

What are the typical features of gout?

There are two phases to gout, each with different radiological patterns (Figs 13.7 & 13.8). In the acute phase, with shedding of crystals in to the joint space, there is an intense inflammatory reaction which may result in:
• Soft tissue swelling
• Joint effusion
• Periarticular osteopenia

The bone remineralizes following control of the acute inflammation and a second, more slowly progressive, chronic tophaceous gout may be seen. The tophi are soft tissue masses that are not aligned with the joint space and the radiology reflects the effects they have on the bone:

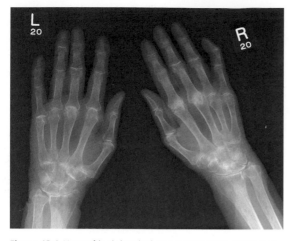

Figure 13.4 X-ray of both hands showing osteopenia and loss of joint space.

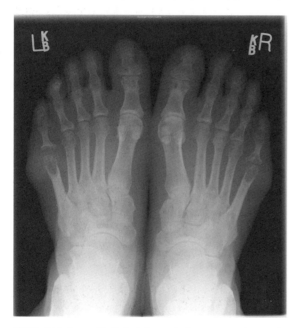

Figure 13.5 X-ray of both feet demonstrating gross erosions and deformity.

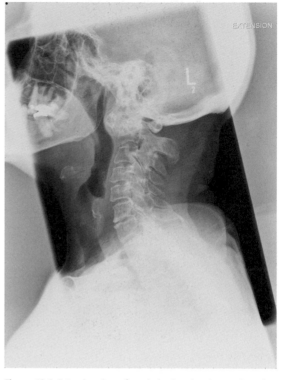

Figure 13.6 Extension view of cervical spine showing erosion of the odontoid peg and C1/2 instability.

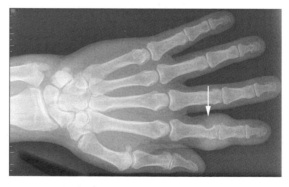

Figure 13.7 X-ray of the right hand shows soft tissue swelling of the index finger with a well-defined erosion of the proximal phalanx away from the joint (arrow).

- Soft tissue mass adjacent to bone (not usually calcified).
- Lace-like response of the adjacent periosteum.
- Well-marginated subchondral cystic rarefactions. These break through the cortex to give erosions with an overhanging edge 'rat-bite' appearance.
- Normal or increased bone density.
- Frank bone destruction in advanced cases.

David returns to see his GP, who explains the plain radiograph report. All the blood tests are normal, consistent with psoriatic arthropathy. The GP refers David to a rheumatologist for further treatment, who agrees with the GP's diagnosis of psoriatic arthritis.

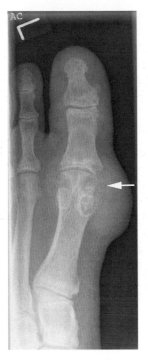

Figure 13.8 X-ray of the left first toe demonstrating a gouty tophus with erosions (arrow).

What treatments might the rheumatologist offer David?

The pain associated with psoriatic arthritis should be treated with appropriate analgesics:

- Paracetamol
- Non-steroidal anti-inflammatory drugs
- Weak opioid drugs

Box 13.4 Side-effects of corticosteroids

- Hypertension
- Diabetes mellitus
- Osteoporosis
- Obesity
- Adrenal suppression
- Immunosuppression
- Thin skin

- Easy bruising
- Stretch marks
- Moon face
- Buffalo hump
- Proximal myopathy
- Avascular necrosis
- Peptic ulcer

These will reduce pain, but have no effect on disease progression. Disease modifying antirheumatic drugs (DMARDs) are used for this:

- Methotrexate
- Azathioprine

When DMARDs fail, patients may be offered anti-TNF-α monoclonal antibody drugs.

Corticosteroids are used as a last resort, for short periods only. This is because of the many significant side-effects of these drugs (Box 13.4).

David is prescribed methotrexate, as well as the simple analgesia he was given by the GP. At a review 6 weeks later, he is found to have made a good clinical recovery and is reviewed annually thereafter by the rheumatologist.

CASE REVIEW

A 30-year-old man with a history of psoriasis (including nail changes) presents to his GP with painful swollen fingers and toes. On examination there is a symmetrical non-deforming polyarthropathy affecting the fingers and toes, with signs of active synovitis.

The GP prescribes analgesia and arranges blood tests and plain X-rays of the hands and feet. The plain X-ray of the hands shows swollen soft tissues. The corresponding X-ray of the feet shows loss of joint space, particularly involving the DIP joints, with acro-osteolysis – typical features of psoriatic arthritis.

The GP refers the patient to a rheumatologist, who agrees with the GP's diagnosis of psoriatic arthritis. The rheumatologist prescribes methotrexate, a DMARD, and follows up the patient 6 weeks later. He makes a good clinical recovery and is reviewed annually thereafter.

KEY POINTS

- The differential for a symmetrical polyarthritis is wide
- Blood tests and plain X-rays play a part in the diagnosis
- Other features in the examination are particularly helpful in making the diagnosis, such as psoriatic plaques
- Most patients developing psoriatic arthritis will have psoriatic nail changes
- Psoriatic arthritis is one of the seronegative arthritides
- Psoriatic arthritis may manifest in one of five ways
- Typical features of psoriatic arthritis on plain X-ray include:
  - DIP joint involvement
  - acro-osteolysis
  - lack of juxta-articular osteopenia
- Typical features of osteoarthritis on plain X-ray include:
  - loss of joint space
  - osteophytes
  - subchondral sclerosis
  - subchondral cysts
- Typical features of rheumatoid arthritis on plain X-ray include:
  - loss of joint space
  - soft tissue swelling
  - juxta-articular osteopenia
  - marginal erosions
  - more deformity than other arthritides (except arthritis mutilans)

A 42-year-old woman with abdominal pain

Jane Pilgrim, a 42-year-old woman, presents to the accident and emergency department with a 4-hour history of severe rapid onset colicky (i.e. coming and going in waves lasting a minute or so) right upper quadrant abdominal pain. She has never had pain like this before. She also complains of nausea. She has no significant past medical, surgical or family history.

What key features would you look for on examination?

Colicky right upper quadrant pain suggests a biliary origin. Jaundice is therefore particularly important to assess for (jaundice is the clinical finding of yellow skin and sclerae, which occurs with a hyperbilirubinaemia of at least 40 mmol/L). The abdomen should be palpated, and the patient should be assessed for Murphy's sign. The clinical Murphy's sign is described in Box 14.1, along with the sonographic equivalent.

The admitting doctor finds moderate right upper quadrant tenderness, but no rebound or percussion tenderness. Murphy's sign is negative and the patient is not jaundiced.

What is the differential diagnosis of right upper quadrant abdominal pain?

Many of the common causes of right upper quadrant pain are biliary.

- Biliary:
  - acute cholecystitis
  - chronic cholecystitis
  - biliary colic
  - ascending cholangitis

- Hepatic:
  - hepatitis (e.g. viral, alcohol, drug related)
  - acute fatty liver (e.g. in pregnancy)
  - hepatic congestion (e.g. heart failure, Budd–Chiari syndrome)
- Appendicitis (an unusual presentation)
- Renal disease:
  - pyelonephritis
  - urolithiasis
  - hydronephrosis
- Cardiac disease
- Right lower lobe pneumonia:
  - lower chest pain can be easily confused with upper abdominal pain

What investigations would you arrange?

With such a wide range of possibilities, a number of investigations would be required:
- A urine dipstick would be useful to assess for renal causes
- Full blood count (FBC) – to look for a raised white cell count to suggest inflammation or infection
- Urea and electrolytes – to assess for renal impairment
- C-reactive protein (CRP) – to look for inflammation or infection
- Liver function tests – these may be abnormal in either hepatic or biliary disease
- A chest X-ray – to look for right lower lobe consolidation
- An electrocardiogram (ECG) – to look for myocardial ischaemia

The admitting doctor prescribes oral analgesia and arranges the above tests. The urine dipstick and ECG are normal. The results of the blood tests are given in Box 14.2. The chest X-ray is shown in Fig. 14.1.

Radiology: Clinical Cases Uncovered. By A. S. Shaw, E. M. Godfrey, A. Singh and T. F. Massoud. Published 2009 by Blackwell Publishing. ISBN 978-1-4051-8474-8.

Box 14.1 Murphy's sign

Both the clinical and sonographic Murphy's sign are said to indicate acute cholecystitis. The sonographic Murphy's sign is more specific, because tenderness can be definitely linked to the gallbladder anatomically

- *Clinical Murphy's sign.* The patient is asked to exhale, the right upper quadrant is then gently palpated during inspiration. If this elicits tenderness (sometimes causing the patient to stop breathing in), but does not if repeated in the left upper quadrant, the patient is said to have Murphy's sign
- *Sonographic Murphy's sign.* This is assessed in the same way except that pressure applied with the ultrasound probe is substituted for palpation. The ultrasound machine can be used to ensure that pressure is applied over the gallbladder

---

Box 14.2 Blood test results

Full blood count – normal
Urea and electrolytes – normal
C-reactive protein – normal
Liver function tests:
- Albumin – 41 g/L (normal range 35–55)
- Bilirubin – 28 µmol/L (normal range 2–17)
- Alanine transaminase – 28 IU/L (normal range 7–56)
- Alkaline phosphatase – 365 IU/L (normal range 20–126)

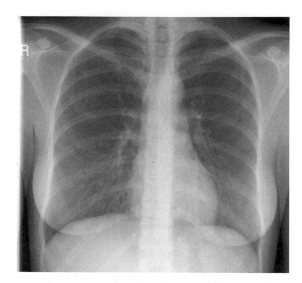

Figure 14.1 Frontal chest X-ray.

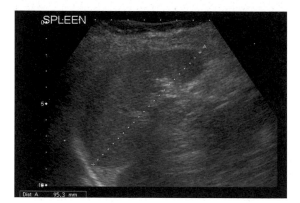

Figure 14.2 Ultrasound of the spleen.

What does the image show?

This is a normal frontal chest X-ray. A typical report might read 'The heart and mediastinum are normal, the lungs and pleural space are clear.'

How do you interpret the blood results?

The blood results show a slight rise in bilirubin. This is below the level that would be detectable clinically as jaundice. The alkaline phosphatase is also raised, suggestive of an obstructive cause of the hyperbilirubinaemia. The remaining blood tests are all normal.

What would you do next?

Biliary obstruction is most simply and cheaply assessed with an ultrasound examination. When assessing the gallbladder with any type of imaging it is crucial that the patient is fasted for at least 4 hours before. This is because any food or fluid (other than water) may induce the release of cholecystokinin, causing contraction of the gallbladder. The contracted gallbladder cannot be assessed for wall thickening, and its contents may be obscured.

Miss Pilgrim is fasted until later that day, at which point she undergoes an ultrasound of the biliary tract.

What do the images show?

Figure 14.2 shows a normal size spleen (any size up to 13 cm is normal for an adult). Figure 14.3 shows the

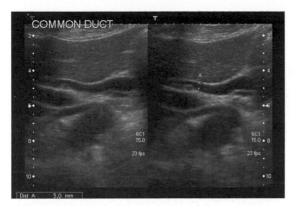

Figure 14.3 Ultrasound of the liver.

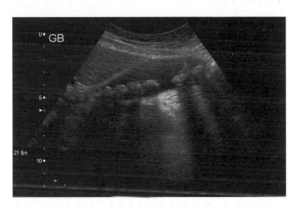

Figure 14.4 Ultrasound of the gallbladder.

common duct which is also normal in size (any size up to 6 mm is normal in adults, an extra 1 mm is allowed for every decade over 50 years). Also shown on the image is the right hepatic artery in cross-section (appearing as a circle) and running parallel to the common duct, the portal vein. Radiologists use the term common duct to refer to both the common bile duct and the common hepatic duct. This is because the cystic duct is often not visible on ultrasound, making the distinction between common bile duct and common hepatic duct impossible.

Figure 14.4 shows the gallbladder. It is filled with multiple echogenic foci that cast acoustic shadows. These two features, coupled with mobility when the patient is rolled on their side, are diagnostic of gallstones. The gallbladder is thin walled and there is no fluid around it, both of which can suggest acute cholecystitis. The report also says that the sonographic Murphy's sign is negative.

What diagnosis is most likely?

The history of colicky right upper abdominal pain, coupled with the blood tests and ultrasound findings would support a diagnosis of biliary colic.

What treatment would you recommend?

Miss Pilgrim should be referred to a hepatobiliary surgeon for consideration of a laparoscopic cholecystectomy. This would make future attacks of biliary colic much less likely (stones can still form within the bile ducts themselves, although this occurs much less frequently than in the gallbladder).

In the meantime the patient should be treated with analgesia. Paracetamol and non-steroidal anti-inflammatory drugs should be given, providing there are no contraindications. The pain is usually severe enough to require opioid analgesia too.

The liver function tests and pain improve over 24 hours. Miss Pilgrim is discharged and referred to a hepatobiliary surgeon. After discussion of the risks and benefits, she is put on the waiting list for a laparoscopic cholecystectomy. Given the history of abnormal liver function tests, an intra-operative cholangiogram (to look for gallstones in the common bile duct) is also planned.

Just over a month later (2 weeks before her planned cholecystectomy), she again presents to the accident and emergency department with abdominal pain. On this occasion, the pain feels very different. It is constant, epigastric and radiates through to the back. She is more nauseated on this occasion and has vomited twice. On examination she has tenderness of the epigastrium and bluish discoloration of the flanks.

What diagnosis do you suspect?

This is a classic history for pancreatitis. Alternatives to consider would be a leaking aortic aneurysm (unlikely at the age of 42) and duodenal or gastric pathology.

What tests would you arrange?

• Amylase – this would be significantly raised in pancreatitis. Lipase is an alternative to amylase that is more sensitive, specific and expensive. It is not available in all centres.

• FBC – raised white cell count would indicate inflammation or infection.

• Urea and electrolytes – to look for associated renal dysfunction.

- CRP – raised in inflammation and infection.
- Liver function tests – to look for associated biliary or hepatic pathology.

The above tests are arranged by the admitting doctor who also prescribes paracetamol, diclofenac and morphine with ondansetron for nausea. He inserts a nasogastric tube and prescribes intravenous fluids.

The blood test results are given below:

Amylase	*1104 U/L (normal range 25–125)*
FBC	*Normal except WCC – 13.4 × 10^9/L (4–11)*
Urea and electrolytes	*Creatinine 165 μmol/L (<115) Urea 7.5 mmol/L (1.2–6.4)*
CRP	*125 mg/L (<5)*
Liver function tests	*Normal except alkaline phosphatase 420 IU/L (20–70)*

Do the blood results support the diagnosis of pancreatitis?

Yes, the amylase is several times above the upper limit of normal. The raised white cell count (WCC) and CRP levels support the diagnosis, indicating an inflammatory response.

What is the likely cause?

Almost half of all pancreatitis is caused by gallstones. In Miss Pilgrim's case, her recent diagnosis with gallstones and biliary colic make this even more likely. A further 25% of cases of pancreatitis are caused by alcohol. Other identifiable causes make up approximately 5%, with the remaining 20% labelled as idiopathic. A well-known mnemonic for remembering the various causes is given in Box 14.3.

Is imaging indicated?

Not at this point. An ultrasound would be indicated if the gallbladder had not been previously imaged. Given Miss Pilgrim has had an ultrasound demonstrating gallstones, a repeat examination is not necessary.

CT has two main roles:

1 In patients where there is doubt over the diagnosis, CT can help by excluding other diagnoses (such as aortic aneurysm) and identifying features of pancreatitis.
2 In patients with an established diagnosis of pancreatitis, CT is useful to identify complications of pancreatitis (e.g. pancreatic necrosis or pseudocyst formation). This

---

Box 14.3 Causes of pancreatitis – GET SMASHED

Gallstones
Ethanol
Trauma
Steroids
Mumps
Autoimmune, e.g. polyarteritis nodosa
Scorpion stings
Hyperlipidaemia/hypercalcaemia
ERCP
Drugs, e.g. azathioprine

---

is best performed at least 4 days after, and ideally 6–10 days after the onset of symptoms. Earlier CT examinations may underestimate the degree of pancreatic necrosis.

What is the point of identifying patients at risk of severe pancreatitis?

Patients with severe pancreatitis are more at risk of developing complications or dying from the disease. They should be managed more aggressively by admitting them to a high dependency unit (HDU) or intensive therapy unit (ITU). In patients with severe gallstone pancreatitis, endoscopic retrograde cholangiopancreatography (ERCP) with sphincterotomy to facilitate passage of gallstones should be undertaken within 72 hours of onset of abdominal pain. Cholecystectomy in these patients should ideally be performed before discharge to prevent recurrent (potentially life-threatening) attacks.

What methods are available for identifying patients at risk of severe pancreatitis?

Up to 4 days after the onset of symptoms, we rely on various clinical and biochemical parameters. After 4 days, CT may be used as an adjunct.

The various predictors of severity include:
- Acute Physiology and Chronic Health Evaluation Score II (APACHE II) of >8. This is useful within the first 24 hours after admission. It is less widely used than the Glasgow Criteria because of its complexity.
- Glasgow Criteria of >2 (Box 14.4). This is useful at 48 hours after admission (not before).

Box 14.4 Severity scoring for pancreatitis: the Modified Glasgow Criteria – PANCREAS

PaO$_2$	<8.6 kPa or 60 mmHg
Age	>55 years
Neutrophils	WCC >15.0 × 10^9/L
Calcium	<2.0 mmol/L
Raised urea	>16 mmol/L
Enzymes	LDH >600 IU/L
Albumin	<32 g/L
Sugar	Glucose >10 mmol/L (assuming no history of diabetes)

Three positive criteria or more makes severe pancreatitis likely. Less than three makes severe pancreatitis unlikely

---

Box 14.5 Balthazar scoring system for CT in acute pancreatitis

Pancreas and peripancreatic tissues

• Normal pancreas	0
• Oedema of pancreas, normal peripancreatic tissues	1
• Mild extrapancreatic soft tissue stranding	2
• Severe extrapancreatic soft tissue stranding with at least 1 collection	3
• Multiple extrapancreatic collections	4

Pancreatic enhancement

• Normal enhancement	0
• Non-enhancement of 1/3 of the pancreas	2
• Non-enhancement of 1/3 to 1/2	4
• Non-enhancement of >1/2	6

Score	Complications	Mortality
0–3	8%	3%
4–6	35%	6%
7–10	92%	17%

- CRP of >150 mg/L. This is useful at 48 hours after admission (not before).
- Organ failure, particularly if persisting for more than 48 hours.
- The Balthazar Severity Score (Box 14.5). This is a scoring system based on CT appearances.

Miss Pilgrim is admitted to the HDU for close monitoring of her fluid balance. She receives aggressive intravenous fluid resuscitation. Her electrolytes are closely monitored. She is provided with a patient-controlled analgesia system for delivering intravenous morphine boluses. She is given supplementary oxygen and a urinary catheter is inserted.

At 48 hours after admission, further blood tests are taken to enable severity scoring according to the Glasgow Criteria. The results are given below:

PaO$_2$ (arterial blood gas on room air)	*11.2 kPa*
Age	*42 years*
WCC	**17.2 × 10^9/L**
Calcium	**1.89 mmol/L**
Urea	*7.4 mmol/L*
Lactate dehydrogenase (LDH)	**784 IU/L**
Albumin	**30 g/L**
Glucose	*7 mmol/L*
CRP	*231 mg/L*
Creatinine	*157 µmol/L*

The parameters that reach the level specified in the Glasgow Criteria are highlighted in bold. This gives a severity score of 4/8, making severe pancreatitis likely. Further evidence that severe pancreatitis is likely is given by the level above 150 mg/L and the continuing renal failure.

What procedure should Miss Pilgrim undergo?

All patients with severe gallstone pancreatitis should ideally undergo ERCP and sphincterotomy within 72 hours of onset of symptoms. This is to allow passage of any obstructing gallstones with the aim of alleviating pressure within the pancreatic duct.

Miss Pilgrim undergoes ERCP with sphincterotomy. The gastroenterologist requests a CT examination for the following day to coincide with 4 days after the onset of symptoms (the earliest appropriate time to perform CT to look for complications of pancreatitis).

What do the images show?

Figure 14.5 shows fluid density in flanks. This is abnormal and is the CT equivalent of Grey–Turner's sign (noted by the admitting doctor as bluish discoloration of the flanks).

Figure 14.6 (arrow) shows a collection of fluid surrounding the pancreas. This is not a pseudocyst as there is no high density rim (often erroneously called rim enhancement). Simple fluid collections can be managed conservatively, providing the patient is making good

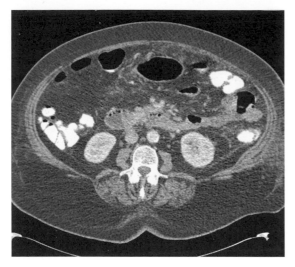

Figure 14.5 Axial CT image through the abdomen.

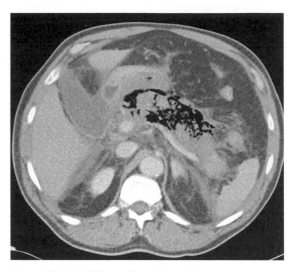

Figure 14.7 Axial CT image through the abdomen.

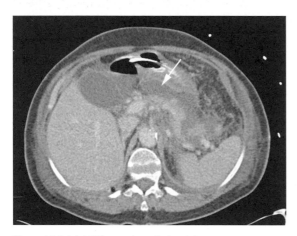

Figure 14.6 Axial CT image through the abdomen.

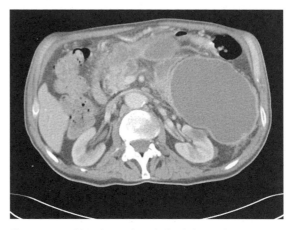

Figure 14.8 Axial CT image through the abdomen demonstrating a pancreatic pseudocyst.

clinical progress. If there is a suspicion of infection, diagnostic aspiration is indicated.

Miss Pilgrim makes steady progress, her renal impairment improves (despite the dose of intravenous contrast medium given for the CT examination) and her CRP falls. Her urinary catheter is removed at day 7.

At 12 days after the onset of abdominal pain, her temperature spikes to 38.9 °C.

You are called to see the patient on the ward. What should you do?

After taking a history and examining the patient, a urine dipstick should be arranged. If positive, a mid-stream urine sample should be sent to the microbiology laboratory. If the urine dipstick is negative, or there are respiratory symptoms or signs, a chest X-ray should be requested. Blood cultures should be taken, as well as samples for FBC and CRP.

The urine dipstick and chest X-ray are both normal. The WCC and CRP have both risen since the previous sample.

What would you do next?

The simple causes having been excluded, the patient should be considered for a repeat CT examination. Given the recent history of severe pancreatitis, there is a risk of intra-abdominal sepsis.

What does the image show?

The image shows gas and fluid within the pancreatic bed. This is almost diagnostic of infected pancreatic necrosis. An uncomplicated pancreatic pseudocyst is shown in Fig. 14.8 for comparison (note the high density rim).

What is the appropriate management?

The patient requires intervention to remove the infected necrotic material from the pancreatic bed. The precise technique is evolving, and depends on local expertise. The options include:

- Open débridement (used less nowadays)
- Percutaneous drainage with large drains inserted radiologically
- Endoscopic drainage using endoscopic ultrasound

Miss Pilgrim underwent open débridement, along with simultaneous open cholecystectomy. She made a slow but uneventful postoperative recovery with the first three postoperative days being spent in ITU. She was discharged 4 weeks after her initial presentation.

CASE REVIEW

Jane Pilgrim, a 42-year-old woman, presents with a history of colicky right upper quadrant abdominal pain. She is not jaundiced clinically. Blood tests reveal a raised alkaline phosphatase and a slightly raised bilirubin. An ultrasound of the biliary tract reveals gallstones but no biliary duct dilatation. A diagnosis of biliary colic is made. She sees a hepatobiliary surgeon and is put on the waiting list for a laparoscopic cholecystectomy.

Two weeks later, while waiting for her operation, Miss Pilgrim develops constant epigastric pain radiating to the back. Initial blood tests reveal a raised amylase, and a diagnosis of pancreatitis is made. Renal impairment is identified via a raised creatinine, and she is therefore admitted to HDU.

Further blood tests, taken 48 hours after the onset of symptoms, identify Miss Pilgrim as being in danger of developing severe pancreatitis. An urgent ERCP with sphincterotomy is therefore arranged.

A CT examination performed 4 days after the onset of symptoms identifies a simple peripancreatic fluid collection. The patient is managed conservatively as she is making good clinical progress.

At 12 days after the onset of symptoms, the patient becomes febrile. The urine dipstick and chest X-ray are clear. A repeat CT examination reveals gas and fluid within the pancreatic bed. Infected pancreatic necrosis is suspected. The patient undergoes open pancreatic débridement and open cholecystectomy, and has an uncomplicated but slow recovery.

KEY POINTS

- Patients presenting with right upper quadrant pain should have blood sent for liver function tests
- Right upper quadrant pain is often assessed with ultrasound
- Pancreatitis is usually a biochemical diagnosis
- CT can be helpful to make the diagnosis of pancreatitis in equivocal cases
- In cases where there is no diagnostic uncertainty, CT can also be used to look for complications, such as pancreatic necrosis or pseudocyst formation
- When looking for complications, CT should be delayed to at least 4 days after the onset of symptoms
- Simple collections of fluid (i.e. without a high density rim) can be managed conservatively if the patient is improving clinically
- A repeat CT should be arranged if the patient's condition deteriorates
- When a ward patient becomes febrile, carry out simple tests first such as a urine dipstick or chest X-ray
- Gas and fluid within the pancreatic bed is highly suggestive of infected pancreatic necrosis
- Infected pancreatic necrosis should be drained

Further reading

UK guidelines for the management of pancreatitis. http://www. bsg.org.uk.

Case 15 A 57-year-old man with jaundice

Cameron Davis, a 57-year-old solicitor, presents to his GP with a 2-day history of jaundice and itching, but no abdominal pain. Mr Davis had been previously fit and well, with no other medical problems and taking no regular medications. On questioning, he reports 'drinking socially', but not to excess.

What potential causes for Mr Davis' jaundice would you consider?

- Acute hepatitis:
  - viral hepatitis (A, B or C)
  - alcohol induced
  - drug reactions
  - Gilbert's syndrome
- Biliary obstruction:
  - gallstones
  - pancreatic tumour
- Chronic liver disease:
  - fibrosis
  - cirrhosis
- Systemic disease:
  - metastases

On examination, Mr Davis is jaundiced. The liver and spleen are just palpable, indicating that there is hepatosplenomegaly. The GP notices spider naevi on Mr Davis' abdomen.

What investigations would you request initially? What information do they give?

The key investigations at this point are as follows:

Radiology: Clinical Cases Uncovered. By A. S. Shaw, E. M. Godfrey, A. Singh and T. F. Massoud. Published 2009 by Blackwell Publishing. ISBN 978-1-4051-8474-8.

1 Liver function tests
- Bilirubin – a marker of severity of jaundice:
- Enzymes – the serum enzymes are raised differentially according to whether the jaundice is secondary to hepatocyte dysfunction (raised aspartate aminotransferase [AST] and alanine aminotransferase [ALT]) or biliary obstruction (raised alkaline phosphatase and gamma glutamyl transferase [GGT])
- Albumin – a marker of synthetic liver function
2 Liver ultrasound
- Evaluate liver parenchyma:
  - smooth/irregular contour
  - echotexture (homogeneous/heterogeneous)
  - are there any focal lesions?
- Evaluate biliary system:
  - are the bile ducts dilated?
- Check vascular patency and flow:
  - are the portal and hepatic veins patent?
- Look for signs of portal hypertension:
  - spleen size
  - ascites

The liver function tests show a mildly elevated bilirubin and reduced albumin indicating poor hepatocyte function. AST, ALT and GGT are all elevated.

What abnormality does this show?

The ultrasound study was reported to be abnormal; an image of the right liver is shown in Fig. 15.1. The black structure seen anteriorly (top of the image) is the normal gallbladder. Superior to this (left of the image) is the liver, which has a heterogeneous (coarse) echotexture in keeping with a cirrhotic liver. Lying posteriorly (bottom left of the image) there is a rounded lesion within the liver which has a dark rim, hence it may be called a 'target lesion' (arrow). This lesion is abutting the right hemidiaphragm (bright white curved line in the bottom left of the image).

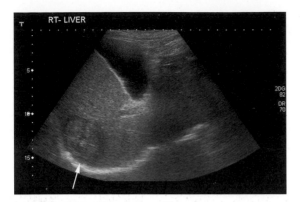

Figure 15.1 Ultrasound image of the right liver.

The ultrasound report states that there is a 5.4cm diameter lesion in the liver which appears to be cirrhotic. The spleen is mildly enlarged but there is no ascites. Mr Davis was referred to a hepatologist for further management.

What does the radiologist mean by 'appears to be cirrhotic'?

Cirrhosis is a histological, not a radiological diagnosis. However, there are a number of features, which may be encountered on various methods of imaging the liver, that indicate that there is cirrhosis and/ or portal hypertension (Box 15.1). These are not particularly sensitive, and cannot differentiate fibrosis from cirrhosis.

What is the lesion likely to represent? What blood test would you request?

Benign lesions such as cysts, haemangiomas, fibrous nodular hyperplasia and adenomas are commonly seen in patients with normal livers, but are rarely encountered in patients with cirrhosis. Metastases from other primary tumours are also seen frequently in patients with a 'normal' underlying liver, but are extremely unusual in the presence of cirrhosis.

The cirrhotic liver constitutes bands of fibrosis with regenerative nodules. Some of these nodules may become dysplastic and these may progress to frank malignancy (hepatocellular carcinoma (hepatoma) [HCC]). Small dysplastic nodules (<2cm) are difficult to differentiate from HCC and hence most guidelines suggest regular surveillance of patients with cirrhosis. This usually comprises 6-monthly ultrasound and serum α-fetoprotein (AFP). The sensitivity of ultrasound in this area is dependent upon several factors, notably operator experience and technique, the equipment used and the body habitus

Box 15.1 Radiological features suggesting cirrhosis and portal hypertension

Cirrhosis
- Irregular contour
- Atrophic liver
- Differential atrophy and hypertrophy of liver segments
- Heterogeneous echotexture (US only)
- Loss of pulsatility in the hepatic veins (US only)

Portal hypertension
- Reversal of blood flow in the portal vein (US only)
- Portosystemic venous shunts (varices)
- Splenomegaly
- Ascites
- Recanalization of the paraumbilical vein

Box 15.2 Hepatocellular carcinoma

- Malignant tumour of hepatocytes
- Usually arises in cirrhotic livers
- Twice as common in men than women
- Patients are usually >40 years of age
- Increasing in incidence
- Fifth most common malignant tumour worldwide
- Highest incidence in countries where viral hepatitis is endemic

of the patient. Serum AFP should not be used alone as many tumours do not secrete AFP. The use of routine surveillance often identifies tumours at an earlier stage when treatment is more likely to be curative. As this lesion is 5.4 cm in diameter, it is almost certainly a HCC (Box 15.2).

The serum AFP was found to be elevated. Mr Davis was referred for a CT to confirm the diagnosis and stage the extent of disease (Figs 15.2–15.4).

What do these images demonstrate?

The lesion in the right side of the liver is not seen without intravenous contrast medium. Enhancement in the arterial phase (Fig. 15.3, arrow) and 'washout' in the portal venous phase is characteristic of HCC. Between the stomach and the aorta is an enhancing structure with a serpiginous shape. These are varices (abnormally dilated veins shunting blood from the portal to the systemic

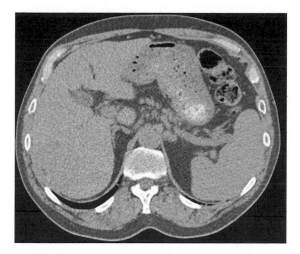

Figure 15.2 Axial CT image through the liver without intravenous contrast medium.

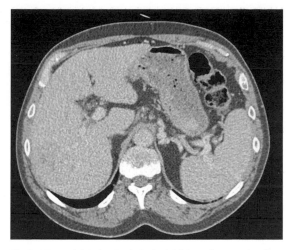

Figure 15.4 Axial CT image through the liver at the same level following intravenous contrast medium in the portal venous phase.

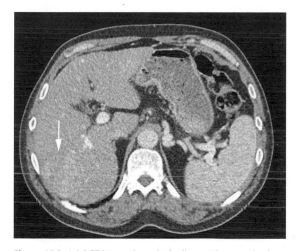

Figure 15.3 Axial CT image through the liver at the same level following intravenous contrast medium in the arterial phase.

venous system, bypassing the liver) and are a sign of portal hypertension.

A number of investigations are performed to try to establish the cause of the underlying liver disease: viral hepatitis screen, autoantibody screen, blood iron and copper levels. All of these proved negative and Mr Davis was again questioned about his alcohol intake. When pressed, he stated that he usually drank half a bottle of wine while entertaining clients each lunch-time and 'a couple of pints of beer after work to relieve stress'.

How many units of alcohol is this and what are considered 'safe' levels?

A single unit of alcohol is equivalent to a single glass (125 mL) of 9% alcohol wine or ½ pint of normal strength beer. When estimating someone's alcohol consumption, it is important to remember that most wine has 12–15% alcohol and is often served in glasses larger than 125 mL. A 750-mL bottle of wine contains approximately 10 units of alcohol. Many 'premium' beers are stronger than average, equivalent to 3 units per pint. Furthermore, a large proportion of people will under-report their alcohol intake when questioned on the matter.

The UK government considers the maximum safe level of alcohol intake to be 28 units/week for a man and 21 units for a woman. However, patients may develop liver disease drinking less than this amount if genetically susceptible.

Mr Davis is diagnosed with cirrhosis secondary to alcohol excess.

Should a biopsy be performed? If so, what should be biopsied?

The background liver may be biopsied to confirm the diagnosis of cirrhosis. This may affect the treatment options available to him. Biopsy of HCC is controversial because of the risk of seeding the tumour along the track of the biopsy needle. This is particularly pertinent when the patient is being considered for transplantation.

Consequently, practice varies from centre to centre with many relying on imaging alone to make the diagnosis and guide further management. When histological confirmation of HCC is not obtained, many centres seek to confirm the diagnosis by visualizing the lesion on two imaging techniques.

What are the treatment options available to Mr Davis?

Several treatment options exist for patients with HCC.
- Liver transplantation:
  - single tumour <5 cm in diameter
  - up to three tumours each measuring <3 cm in diameter
  - patients with alcohol-induced cirrhosis need to be abstinent for 6 months
  - other indications and contraindications for liver transplantation are given in Box 15.3
- Liver resection:
  - usually primarily in non-cirrhotic patients because of insufficient reserve
- Radiofrequency (or microwave) ablation:
  - direct application of energy to the tumour via a probe
  - heats the tumour to cause necrosis
  - most effective with small tumours (<5 cm diameter), but multiple treatments can be used for large tumours
- Arterial embolization:
  - percutaneous catheter inserted via femoral artery
  - embolic material injected in to hepatic artery branches
  - may be combined with chemotherapy
  - requires patent portal vein
- Chemotherapy:
  - gives a small survival benefit, but not curative

In view of the lesion size and the underlying cirrhosis, Mr Davis was referred for transarterial chemoembolization (Figs 15.5–15.7) of the HCC but wishes to know what the procedure involves.

What should you tell him?
- He will be sedated for the procedure
- A small catheter will be inserted via his femoral artery
- The chemotherapy agent will be injected in to the small arteries feeding the tumour, usually coated on small particles which will block off the feeding blood vessels
- Mr Davis will feel some discomfort and have 'flu-like' symptoms for in the first 10–14 days after the procedure, but that this will gradually improve
- The procedure may need to be repeated to complete therapy
- The risks of the procedure include bruising, vascular injury and infection

Two weeks after the procedure, Mr Davis presented to the hepatology team with abdominal pain and a fever. A CT of the abdomen is performed to evaluate the liver (Figs 15.8 & 15.9).

What does the CT image show?

At the site of the tumour in the right liver there is no longer any enhancement. Within the centre of the tumour there are several discrete pockets of gas (black areas). This indicates that an abscess has formed within the necrotic tumour.

The abscess was treated by percutaneous drainage and a course of antibiotics. Three months later, Mr Davis re-presented to the hepatology team with a swelling over the site where the abscess drainage had been performed.

Box 15.3 Clinical indications for liver transplantation

Acute liver failure
Variable depending on the aetiology, important features include:
- pH <7.3
- Prothrombin time (PT) >100 seconds or INR >6.5
- Grade 3–4 encephalopathy

Chronic liver disease
- Bilirubin 6 mg/dL (170 μmol/L)
- Deteriorating synthetic function (serum albumin <30 g/L, unrelated to active infection)
- Refractory ascites
- Recurrent spontaneous bacterial peritonitis
- Recurrent bacterial cholangitis
- Recurring encephalopathy
- Hepatopulmonary syndrome
- Hepatic osteodystrophy
- Poor quality of life (e.g. extreme fatigue, intractable pruritus)

Hepatocellular carcinoma
- 1 lesion <5 cm in diameter
- Up to 3 lesions, each <3 cm in diameter

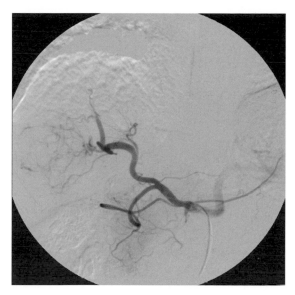

Figure 15.5 Early arterial phase image from an hepatic artery angiogram with the catheter tip in the common hepatic artery.

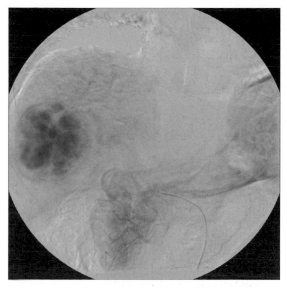

Figure 15.7 Parenchymal phase image from an hepatic artery angiogram. Abnormal enhancement of the right liver lesion is clearly seen.

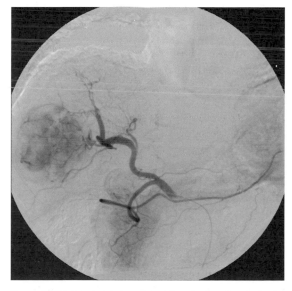

Figure 15.6 Late arterial phase image from an hepatic artery angiogram. Abnormal tumour circulation can be seen in the right liver.

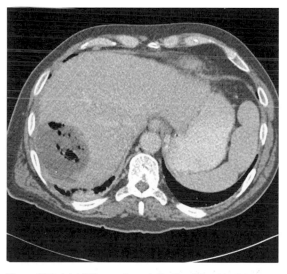

Figure 15.8 Axial CT image through the liver following the administration of intravenous contrast medium.

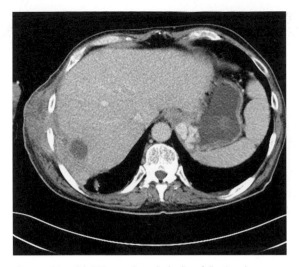

Figure 15.9 Axial CT image through the liver following the administration of intravenous contrast medium.

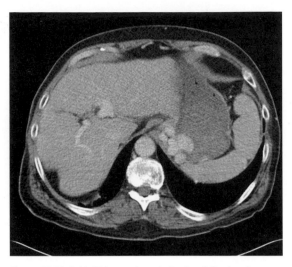

Figure 15.10 Axial CT image through the liver following the administration of intravenous contrast medium 1 month after radiotherapy demonstrating resolution of the tumour mass.

What is the cause of the right-sided swelling?

There is abnormal soft tissue in the muscles and subcutaneous tissues on the right side of the abdominal wall. A tongue of tissue of similar density can be seen extending through the liver to the small low density area which represents the treated abscess. There are no pockets of gas or fluid within this mass. The features indicate that residual tumour within the abscess site has tracked (seeded) along the drain site and is now growing in the subcutaneous tissues.

Mr Davis' tumour recurrence was treated with a course of radiotherapy and the mass resolved (Fig. 15.10).

CASE REVIEW

Cameron Davis, a 57-year-old solicitor, presented to his GP with a short history of jaundice, the cause for which was unclear. However, on examination there were stigmata of chronic liver disease. An ultrasound examination of his liver revealed that it had an abnormal architecture and identified a 5.4-cm focal lesion. Mr Davis went on to have a CT study; this confirmed the presence of a large hepatocellular carcinoma in a cirrhotic liver with evidence of portal hypertension. When questioned more closely, Mr Davis' alcohol intake appeared to be the most likely cause of the underlying cirrhosis. The size of the lesion and the underlying chronic liver disease meant that transarterial chemoembolization was considered the most appropriate course of treatment.

Unfortunately, Mr Davis developed an abscess within the necrotic tumour following the procedure. This required percutaneous drainage and a course of antibiotics. Mr Davis re-presented a few months later with a right-sided mass, shown at CT to be recurrent tumour seeding along the drainage track. This recurrence was treated with radiotherapy and the mass resolved.

KEY POINTS

- A patient presenting with jaundice may have biliary obstruction, acute hepatitis, chronic liver disease or systemic disease
- There are numerous causes for cirrhosis and an exhaustive search should be made for the cause
- Patients will often under-report their alcohol intake
- Many patients with cirrhosis present late in the course of the disease when the liver decompensates
- HCC is the fifth most common malignant tumour worldwide

- HCC develops via regenerative and then dysplastic nodules
- Metastases and benign lesions other than regenerative or dysplastic nodules are very uncommon in cirrhotic livers
- Patients at risk of developing HCC should undergo regular screening with ultrasound and serum AFP
- Screening enables earlier detection of tumours, is more likely to identify smaller tumours and hence means that cure is more likely

Case 16   A 23-year-old woman with diarrhoea

Gale Morland, a 23-year-old woman presents to her GP with a 1-month history of intermittent central abdominal pain. She also describes an increase in stool frequency such that she has to go to the toilet 4–5 times each day, and always has loose stools. On further questioning, the GP establishes that she has lost about 5 kg in weight unintentionally over the last month. She has no significant past medical history or family history.

On examination she has mild right iliac fossa tenderness but there is no guarding, rebound or percussion tenderness. The bowel sounds are normal.

What differential diagnosis would you consider at this point?

The combination of abdominal pain with diarrhoea raises several possibilities:

- Bowel pathology:
  - gastroenteritis
  - irritable bowel syndrome
  - coeliac disease
  - inflammatory bowel disease
  - malignancy
- Pancreatic insufficiency:
  - cystic fibrosis
  - pancreatitis
- Hyperthyroidism

Although irritable bowel syndrome and gastroenteritis are the most common causes of these symptoms, the former does not usually result in any weight loss, while most cases of gastroenteritis are short-lived and self-limiting. The unintentional weight loss is a particular concern and should prompt further urgent investigations.

Radiology: Clinical Cases Uncovered. By A. S. Shaw, E. M. Godfrey, A. Singh and T. F. Massoud. Published 2009 by Blackwell Publishing. ISBN 978-1-4051-8474-8.

Given the pain in the right iliac fossa, is appendicitis a possibility here?

This is an important decision – if the patient could have appendicitis, he/she should be referred to hospital for review by a surgeon. However, Miss Morland has been symptomatic for a month which makes appendicitis very unlikely. Furthermore, in most (although not all) cases of appendicitis, there are clinical features of peritoneal inflammation such as percussion tenderness.

What initial tests would you arrange?

- Full blood count – to look for a raised white cell count or anaemia (for example, from coeliac disease)
- Urea and electrolytes – to look for evidence of dehydration or electrolyte disturbance
- C-reactive protein (CRP) – to look for evidence of an inflammatory process
- Thyroid function tests – to assess thyroid status
- Stool culture – to look for bacterial causes of gastroenteritis

Gale was asked to return in a week for the results of the tests. The full blood count and CRP were abnormal (Box 16.1). The remaining investigations were all reported as normal.

What do the blood tests show?

There is an inflammatory response, indicated by the raised white cell count and CRP. Furthermore, there is a macrocytic anaemia (low haemoglobin with abnormally large erythrocytes).

What are the causes of a macrocytic anaemia?

Possible causes of a macrocytic anaemia include:

- Vitamin B_{12} deficiency:
  - Crohn's disease
  - pernicious anaemia
  - dietary deficiency

Box 16.1 Full blood count and CRP

Haemoglobin 10.1 g/dL (normal range 13–17)
White cells 14.3 × 10⁹/L (4–11)
Platelets 358 × 10⁹/L (150–400)
Mean corpuscular volume 104.5 fL (80–100)
CRP 100 mg/L (0–5)

Box 16.2 Absorption of iron, vitamin B₁₂ and folate from the gastrointestinal tract

Stomach	Secretes intrinsic factor in to the lumen which binds vitamin B₁₂ to promote absorption
Duodenum	Site of iron absorption
Jejenum	Site of folate absorption
Ileum	Site of vitamin B₁₂–intrinsic factor complex absorption

---

- Folate deficiency:
  - coeliac disease
  - dietary deficiency
- Drugs:
  - methotrexate
  - azathioprine
- Hypothyroidism
- Alcohol excess

Gale denies a history of alcohol excess and is not taking any medication. As we have already seen, her thyroid function tests are normal.

Are there any other blood tests you would request at this point?

Given the macrocytic anaemia, the GP requested vitamin B₁₂ and folate levels. Determining the cause of the anaemia should provide clues as to the likely site of disease (Box 16.2). This will guide further investigations toward either pernicious anaemia (Box 16.3) or coeliac disease (Box 16.4).

The blood tests show vitamin B₁₂ deficiency but normal folate levels. The GP starts Gale on oral vitamin B₁₂ and refers her to a gastroenterologist. The gastroenterologist performs an upper gastrointestinal endoscopy and takes gastric and jejunal biopsies. He also requests a barium small bowel enema and sends blood samples to the immunology

---

Box 16.3 Pernicious anaemia

- Autoantibodies directed against intrinsic factor, and the cells that produce it (gastric parietal cells) result in a condition known as atrophic gastritis
- Intrinsic factor is required for the effective absorption of vitamin B₁₂, and the reduction in intrinsic factor production in atrophic gastritis leads to B₁₂ deficiency – in this context known as pernicious anaemia
- Atrophic gastritis is usually confirmed via upper gastrointestinal endoscopy with biopsies of the stomach
- Autoantibodies such as antiparietal cell and anti-intrinsic factor may be raised, but they are not highly specific
- A Schilling test using radiolabelled B₁₂ can be used to confirm pernicious anaemia, but in practice, this is rarely required in the context of atrophic gastritis
- The treatment for pernicious anaemia is vitamin B₁₂ supplementation, either orally or by intramuscular injection
- Patients with pernicious anaemia (and therefore atrophic gastritis) are predisposed to developing gastric cancer and lymphoma

---

Box 16.4 Coeliac disease

- In genetically susceptible individuals exposed to gliadin-containing foods (such as wheat), an autoimmune reaction occurs against the small bowel mucosa
- The effects are most pronounced in the jejunum, but the whole of the small bowel is affected to some degree
- The gold standard test is an upper gastrointestinal endoscopy with jejunal biopsies
- Autoantibodies such as anti-endomysial and anti-transglutaminase are highly specific but not very sensitive for coeliac disease
- The only treatment is a gluten-free diet
- Patients are at an increased risk of small bowel adenocarcinoma and lymphoma

---

department for anti-endomysial and anti-transglutaminase antibody levels.

What is a barium small bowel enema, and what are the other types of fluoroscopic examination?

Fluoroscopic examinations ('barium' examinations) may be used to assess the entire length of the gastrointestinal tract in a variety of contexts. Usually, barium sulphate compounds are used, but iodine-based water-soluble contrast media are substituted if there are concerns regarding bowel obstruction or perforation.

Starting at the top and working down:

• *Barium swallow.* Assesses the oesophagus: good for functional problems such as achalasia.

• *Barium meal.* To look at the stomach and duodenum. This has been superseded by endoscopy which is much more accurate, and enables both biopsy and treatment.

• *Barium follow through.* To visualize the small bowel. The patient drinks the barium solution and images of the small bowel are obtained as it passes through.

• *Barium small bowel enema (also known as enteroclysis).* This test is also used in small bowel disorders. Instead of being ingested, the barium solution is instilled via a naso-jejunal tube. As there is a continuous column of barium distending the small bowel, the images are better than a follow-through and enables depiction of more subtle abnormalities. However, the insertion of a nasojejunal tube means that this is less pleasant for the patient.

• *Barium enema.* Barium and air are instilled via a rectal tube to look at the colon and rectum. This has being increasingly replaced by colonoscopy or CT colono-graphy in many centres and is a poor third to these examinations.

What do the images show? What is the likely diagnosis?

In Fig. 16.1, the nasojejunal tube is seen superiorly lying with its tip in the proximal jejunum with barium having passed through the small bowel to reach the caecum inferiorly on the right. Normal loops of small bowel are seen superiorly and to the left. Adjacent to the caecum there is a segment of abnormal ileum. The abnormal area of bowel shows luminal narrowing (it does not open out fully), irregular mucosa (indicating ulceration) and wall thickening (there are no other loops seen immediately next to it). In the magnified view (Fig. 16.2), the area of abnormality can be seen more clearly.

The combination of mucosal ulceration, strictures, wall thickening and alternating normal and abnormal bowel segments is characteristic of Crohn's disease. This most commonly affects the terminal ileum and therefore the features all point to this being the underlying cause. In the differential diagnosis one might also consider tuberculosis, although this would be very unusual in the absence of risk factors such as immunosuppression or a history of travel to an area with endemic tuberculosis.

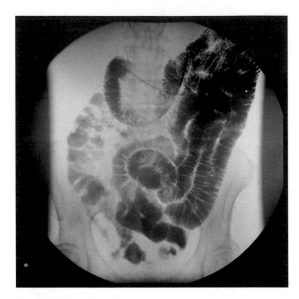

Figure 16.1 Small bowel enema study image.

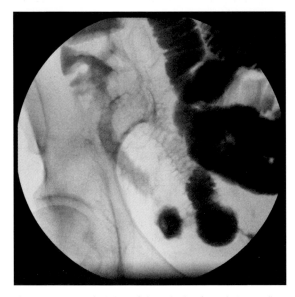

Figure 16.2 Magnified view of the right iliac fossa during small bowel enema.

Yersinia is a common infective cause of terminal ileitis but would not cause stenosis, ulceration or skip lesions.

Why and how should this be confirmed?

The treatment for Crohn's disease can have significant side-effects and will potentially need to be continued for many years. Furthermore, a diagnosis of Crohn's disease will have a major effect on the patient's life: for example,

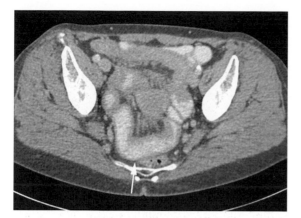

Figure 16.3 Axial CT image through the abdomen.

he/she may find it more difficult to obtain life or medical insurance. It is therefore essential to confirm the diagnosis histologically whenever possible. Biopsies are taken endoscopically from any involved site, most commonly the terminal ileum via colonoscopy.

Gale is seen again by the gastroenterologist, who explains the small bowel enema findings. He arranges a colonoscopy. The endoscopist obtains good views of the entire colon which appears normal apart from a thickened ileocaecal valve (typical of Crohn's disease). The terminal ileum is intubated and biopsied, with histology confirming the diagnosis of Crohn's disease.

What similarities and differences are there between Crohn's disease and ulcerative colitis?

There are a number of overlapping features that may make initial diagnosis difficult, particularly in Crohn's disease of the large bowel. A comprehensive comparison is given in Box 16.5.

Gale is started on a course of oral prednisolone and given a 1-month follow-up appointment to see the gastroenterologist. However, 2 weeks later she presents to the accident and emergency department with a 1-day history of severe right iliac fossa pain. Gale's temperature, CRP and white cell count are all raised. An abdominal CT examination is requested by the clinical team.

What do the images show?

The image shows a loop of small bowel with thickened wall (Fig. 16.3, arrow). The loop is associated with prom-

Box 16.5 Crohn's disease vs ulcerative colitis	
Crohn's disease	
Prevalence	30–50/100,000
M/F	Slightly more common in women
Pathology	Transmural inflammation with non-caseating granulomas anywhere from the mouth to the anus, skip lesions
Age	Bimodal onset at 15–30 or 60–70 years
Typical patterns of involvement	Ileocaecal (most common), perianal, multiple segments of small bowel, Crohn's colitis
Radiological appearance	Wall thickening, rosethorn ulcers, cobblestone mucosa, skip lesions, string sign (stenosed lumen), fistulation
Colorectal cancer risk	Increased, but not as much as in ulcerative colitis
Smoking	Increases risk
Ulcerative colitis	
Prevalence	80/100,000
M/F	M = F
Pathology	Crypt inflammation and abscesses
Age	Bimodal onset at 15–30 or 60–70 years
Typical patterns of involvement	Progresses proximally from rectum (rectum spared in only 4%), extends variably. Can involve the entire colon (pancolitis) with backwash ileitis
Radiological appearance	Dilated colon with pseudopolyps, wall thickening
Colorectal cancer risk	Much higher than general and higher than Crohn's disease, particularly if the whole colon is involved
Smoking	Reduces risk

inent mesenteric blood vessels (sometimes called the 'comb' sign). This implies increased vascularity in the region secondary to inflammation. There is no abscess, fluid or free gas demonstrated.

The CT findings, coupled with a raised temperature and inflammatory markers, indicate that Gale has an acute flare-up of Crohn's disease.

> **Box 16.6 Extraintestinal conditions associated with inflammatory bowel disease**
>
> **Hepatobiliary**
> - Gallstones
> - Primary sclerosing cholangitis (1% of Crohn's, 5% of ulcerative colitis)
> - Cholangiocarcinoma
>
> **Renal**
> - Calculi
>   Musculoskeletal
> - Seronegative migratory distal arthropathy (correlates with disease severity)
> - Ankylosing spondylitis-like arthropathy (unrelated to disease severity)
>
> **Eyes**
> - Uveitis
> - Iritis
>
> **Skin**
> - Erythema nodosum
> - Pyoderma gangrenosum
>
> **Other**
> - Digital clubbing

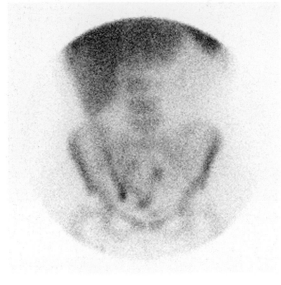

Figure 16.4 Radiolabelled white cell scintigram showing a linear area of increased tracer uptake in the right iliac fossa consistent with an inflamed loop of bowel.

Are there any other imaging modalities that might be useful in this situation?

In the context of an acute abdomen, CT is generally the best initial imaging modality. For monitoring of disease activity and distribution, a radiolabelled white cell scintigram can be used. This will give a physiological map of bowel inflammation (Fig. 16.4). To gain more anatomical information (e.g. to diagnose strictures in a symptomatic patient with Crohn's disease), small bowel enema or follow through is useful. Given the chronic nature of Crohn's disease, many patients will require several examinations throughout their lives. Because these patients are already at an increased risk of colorectal cancer, there is a concern over the cumulative radiation burden. In some centres, magnetic resonance enteroclysis or enterography are being used in place of the small bowel enema and follow through, respectively, this being free from ionizing radiation. Examples of these can be seen in Figs 16.5 and 16.6.

What are the treatment options?

The management of Crohn's may be divided in to medical and surgical categories:
- Lifestyle and dietary:
  - smoking cessation

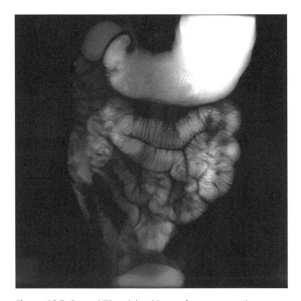

Figure 16.5 Coronal T2-weighted image from a magnetic resonance enteroclysis study with luminal narrowing and loop separation seen in the right iliac fossa.

  - adequate hydration
  - elemental diet (Box 16.7)
- Medical:
  - anti-inflammatory agents (aminosalicylates)
  - corticosteroids (oral or IV, usually for short periods because of side-effects)

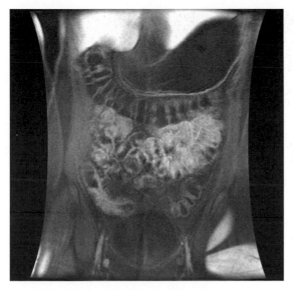

Figure 16.6 Contrast enhanced T1-weighted coronal image from the same study demonstrating thickened bowel wall in the terminal ileum.

○ immune modulators (e.g. azathioprine)
○ monoclonal antibodies (e.g. infliximab)
• Surgical:
○ resection of diseased bowel
○ strictureplasty
○ Seton insertion or laying open of perianal fistulae

Would early surgery be advisable to try and reduce complications?

Crohn's disease cannot be cured by surgical resection. Indeed, Crohn's disease has a propensity to recur at the

> **Box 16.7 Elemental diet**
>
> An elemental diet is a diet that proposes the ingestion, or, in more severe cases, use of a gastric feeding tube of liquidized nutrients, already in a digested form. It is usually composed of amino acids, fats, sugars, vitamins and minerals. However, this diet lacks whole or partial protein, because of its ability to cause an allergic reaction in some people. This diet is used in patients with Crohn's disease so that their inflamed gastrointestinal tract does not have to digest food and has time to heal and begin remission. Elemental diet is usually reserved for severe cases; many patients find it unpleasant and are unwilling to take it.

site of surgical anastamoses and lead to further strictures. Furthermore, healing of wounds is often delayed by the concurrent medication which predisposes the patient to infection and the formation of fistulae. Thus, surgical intervention should be carefully considered. Indications for surgery include the treatment of symptomatic strictures, fistulae and failure of medical therapy. Any resection should remove the shortest possible length of bowel in order that malabsorption from short bowel syndrome may be avoided.

Gale was then reviewed by a gastroenterologist. Given the acute flare up despite steroid therapy, a monoclonal antibody and salicylate were prescribed. Gale made a good recovery and was discharged home.

CASE REVIEW

Gale Morland, a 23-year-old woman, presents to her GP with a 1-month history of central abdominal pain, diarrhoea and weight loss. Following initial investigations, her GP diagnoses macrocytic anaemia caused by vitamin B_{12} deficiency. He starts Gale on oral vitamin B_{12} and refers her to a gastroenterologist.

The gastroenterologist performs an upper gastrointestinal endoscopy, taking gastric and jejunal biopsies to look for atrophic gastritis and coeliac disease, respectively. They also request a barium small bowel enema which demonstrates typical features of Crohn's disease. A colonoscopy

is performed and ileal biopsies confirm Crohn's disease. Gale is treated with a course of oral corticosteroids and outpatient follow-up is arranged.

Prior to her appointment, Gale attends the accident and emergency department with a 1-day history of severe right iliac fossa pain. An abdominal CT examination shows severe inflammation of the distal small bowel, but no evidence of bowel perforation or other indications for surgery. Gale is commenced on anti-inflammatory agents and a monoclonal antibody, making a good recovery.

KEY POINTS

- Unintentional weight loss is a concerning symptom that requires investigation
- Macrocytic anaemia has a variety of causes including folate and vitamin B_{12} deficiency
- The small bowel may be imaged using barium studies. Small bowel enema provides better images than small bowel follow through, but is less pleasant for the patient as it requires nasojejunal intubation
- Typical radiological features of Crohn's disease include strictures, skip lesions, bowel wall thickening, ulceration, cobblestone mucosa (criss-crossing longitudinal and transverse ulcers separated by areas of oedema) and fistulae

- The diagnosis of Crohn's disease may be suggested by imaging, but should ideally be confirmed with histology
- In a patient with Crohn's disease and an acute abdomen, a CT examination is the best imaging test. This will exclude other causes of an acute abdomen and will evaluate potential complications of Crohn's disease
- There are a variety of lifestyle, dietary, medical and surgical approaches available for the treatment of Crohn's disease
- Magnetic resonance enterography and enteroclysis are increasingly used to image patients with Crohn's disease to reduce the cumulative dose of radiation these patients are exposed to

Case 17 — A 67-year-old man with rectal bleeding

John Knight presented to his GP with a 3-month history of rectal bleeding 'on and off' and said that he thought he had 'piles'. The bleeding had started rather abruptly and was bright red, and was accompanied with some discomfort. On questioning, Mr Knight said that he often felt fullness in his rectum, but had no weight loss. A 67-year-old retired policeman, Mr Knight had no previous medical history of note and took no regular medications. On inspection of the perineum, the GP found prominent haemorrhoids and referred Mr Knight to a colorectal surgeon for further management. The surgeon saw Mr Knight and confirmed the GP's findings.

What would you do now?

A digital rectal examination is mandatory in all cases of rectal bleeding to exclude rectal pathology as the cause of bleeding. One should not simply assume that the haemorrhoids are the cause of the bleeding, hence the old surgical adage 'if you don't put your finger in it, you'll put your foot in it.'

Digital rectal examination is uncomfortable for Mr Knight, but the surgeon feels an irregular mass in the rectum. She proceeds to a rigid sigmoidoscopy in the outpatient clinic, visualizes what appears to be tumour and takes a biopsy.

What further investigations are needed at this stage?

• MRI of the rectum – to assess the local stage of disease (Box 17.1)
• Colonoscopy – to assess the remainder of the colon for synchronous tumours
• CT – to evaluate the thorax, abdomen and pelvis for metastases

---

Radiology: Clinical Cases Uncovered. By A. S. Shaw, E. M. Godfrey, A. Singh and T. F. Massoud. Published 2009 by Blackwell Publishing. ISBN 978-1-4051-8474-8.

What do the images show?

To orientate oneself on the sagittal image (Fig. 17.1), one can see the pubic bone on the left of the image and the sacrum on the right. Lying behind the pubic bone is the normal prostate gland with the (almost empty) bladder above it. Behind these structures lies the rectum. The rectum is a tubular structure and therefore should be seen as just an anterior and posterior wall on this view. However, lying between the bladder and the second and third sacral segments there is a large tumour of the upper rectum (Fig. 17.1, arrow). The tumour has mixed signal, but can be seen extending posteriorly from the rectum just anterior to the sacrum. A cross-section through the upper rectum in Fig. 17.2 demonstrates the irregular nature of the tumour mass as it extends out in to the mesorectum.

The mesorectum is an extraperitoneal compartment within the pelvis which contains the rectum and its surrounding fat. It is enclosed by the mesorectal fascia circumferentially, the peritoneal reflection superiorly, and the levator ani muscles inferiorly. It is of crucial importance in rectal cancer as the surgeon will aim to take the mesorectum out in one piece, fascial planes intact (total mesorectal excision). If the tumour extends close to or, as in this case, involves these circumferential resection margins, then surgery is deferred until the tumour can be downsized by chemotherapy or radiotherapy.

Three days later, Mr Knight attends for his colonoscopy. Having negotiated the rectal mass, the operator is unable to progress beyond the sigmoid colon because of its tortuous course.

What other options are available to you to evaluate the proximal colon?

1 *CT colonography.* This is the best radiological method of evaluating the colon (Box 17.2), and could be performed immediately as the patient will have already taken purgatives prior to his colonoscopy.

Box 17.1 MRI of the rectum

- Best method of locally staging invasive rectal cancer
- Uses T2-weighted images of the whole pelvis with targeted high resolution views of the rectum in the sagittal plane and axial oblique plane (perpendicular to the line of the rectum)
- Differentiates stage T2, 3 or 4 disease, but not very early cancer
- Accurately predicts whether the circumferential resection margin is threatened or involved by tumour
- Determines the relationship of the tumour to the sphincter complex inferiorly
- Can identify large vessel invasion by tumour
- Identifies lymph nodes, but is not able to predict reliably which are involved with tumour and which are reactive

Box 17.2 CT colonography

- The patient may be given either purgatives, oral contrast medium, or a combination of the two according to local practice
- The use of oral contrast medium is termed 'faecal tagging'
- The patient follows a low residue diet for 2 days
- For the examination, a rectal tube is inserted and intravenous hyoscine butylbromide (Buscopan) administered
- The colon is insufflated with gas (preferably CO_2)
- The patient is imaged in both the prone and supine positions. This helps to ensure that polyps are not obscured by faeces, fluid or collapsed segments of bowel
- Intravenous contrast medium is administered for symptomatic patients, but not in the screening population
- Images are reviewed on a dedicated workstation and may be presented in a variety of ways, including two-dimensional multiplanar reconstructions, three-dimensional endoluminal views or even with the colon opened out as a 'virtual dissection'
- Most studies report colonography is slightly inferior to colonoscopy, but both perform significantly better than barium enema

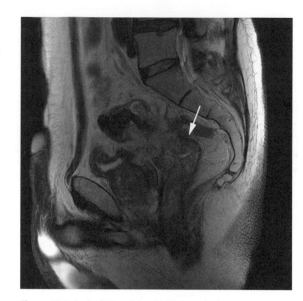

Figure 17.1 Sagittal T2-weighted MRI through the rectum.

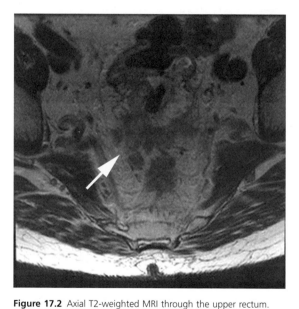

Figure 17.2 Axial T2-weighted MRI through the upper rectum.

2 *'Standard' CT of the abdomen and pelvis.* The patient is given oral contrast medium for 24 hours to opacify the large bowel. This would enable detection of large lesions but has poor sensitivity for polyps and smaller lesions. Both this and the CT colonography could be combined with a CT of the thorax to complete disease staging.

3 *Barium enema.* Fluoroscopic evaluation of the colon is inferior to CT colonography and has thus largely fallen out of favour.

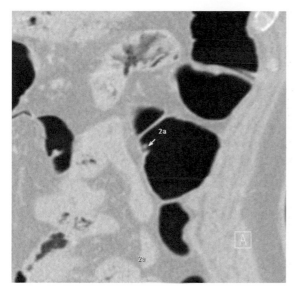

Figure 17.3 Two-dimensional coronal CT colonography image of the descending colon.

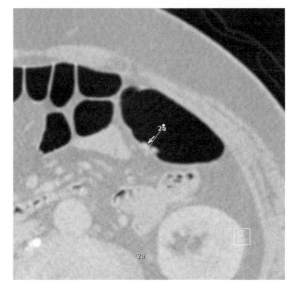

Figure 17.4 Two-dimensional axial CT colonography image of the descending colon.

The endoscopist discusses the case with the radiologist and Mr Knight undergoes a CT colonography and a CT thorax directly from the endoscopy suite.

The CT colonography (Figs 17.3–17.5) is reported to show a small (4 mm) polyp in the descending colon, but is otherwise normal. Polyps less than 1 cm in size are rarely of significance and thus it is decided to follow this up at a later date. The CT study does not demonstrate any metastatic disease in the thorax and abdomen.

The results of the rectal biopsy confirm the diagnosis of a mucinous adenocarcinoma of the rectum. Mr Knight undergoes a course of chemotherapy and radiotherapy and then has a further MRI study of the rectum to assess response and enable surgical planning.

How do these images compare with the initial MRI study?

There has been a marked reduction in the extent of tumour. On the sagittal image (Fig. 17.6), one can see the tumour posterior to the rectum has almost completely resolved. This is confirmed on the axial image (Fig. 17.7) which demonstrates the mass to have reduced and meso-rectal fascia (circumferential resection margins) to be clear of disease.

Mr Knight undergoes an anterior resection to resect the tumour. This means he will have a total mesorectal excision and a primary anastamosis of the two cut ends of colon low

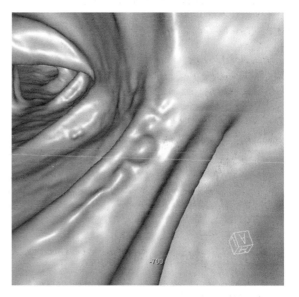

Figure 17.5 Three-dimensional reconstruction showing an endoluminal view of the descending colon.

within the pelvis, just above the sphincter complex, thus avoiding a colostomy.

The procedure passes uneventfully and the surgical histology reports complete excision with the resection margins clear of disease. The surgeon asks you to organize routine surveillance for Mr Knight.

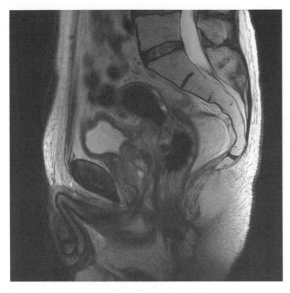

Figure 17.6 Sagittal T2-weighted MRI through the rectum.

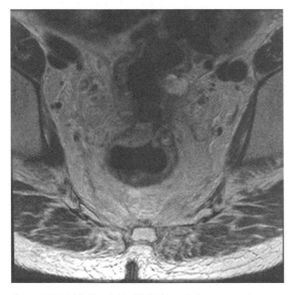

Figure 17.7 Axial T2-weighted MRI through the upper rectum.

What surveillance should Mr Knight undergo?

1 *Colonic.* Mr Knight has not yet had a formal colonoscopy. This should ideally be performed within a few months of the surgery to ensure that the tiny polyp seen on colonoscopy is benign and that there are no other

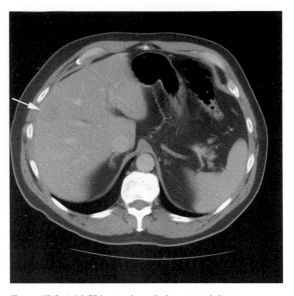

Figure 17.8 Axial CT image through the upper abdomen following administration of intravenous contrast medium.

lesions that have been overlooked. Thereafter, routine colonoscopy should be performed every few years.

2 *Whole body.* Follow-up CT of the chest, abdomen and pelvis should be performed at regular intervals for the first 3 years. The aim is to identify early those patients who develop metastases in order that they may be treated early to improve survival.

Mr Knight had a normal follow-up CT study at 6 months. However, at 12 months, an abnormality was identified on the surveillance CT (Fig. 17.8).

What abnormality is shown on the image?

The image has been acquired in the portal venous phase, approximately 70 seconds following the injection of intravenous contrast medium. In the right liver, there is a focal area of reduced attenuation (Fig. 17.8, arrow). It measures 3.5 cm in diameter. Given the clinical history and the development of a new lesion, this almost certainly represents a metastatic deposit from the rectal tumour.

What therapeutic options would you consider?

• *Surgery.* If all of the metastatic disease can be removed surgically, this will have the best long-term results.

Box 17.3 Radiofrequency ablation

- The patient is either heavily sedated or anaesthetized
- An electrode is placed into the tumour under imaging guidance
- An alternating electrical current is passed through the probe in the radiofrequency spectrum (460–500 kHz)
- The high resistance of the bodily tissues to the electrical current causes local ionic agitation and heating
- Temperatures over 50 °C will result in tissue coagulation
- A single probe will produce coagulation necrosis over a diameter of approximately 3 cm
- Advances in probe design and the use of multiple probes have resulted in larger treatment zones
- Incomplete treatment may occur near to blood vessels as the flowing blood acts as a coolant and prevents tissue necrosis
- Thermal injury may occur to the biliary tree, gallbladder or colon
- Radiofrequency ablation may also be performed on lung, renal or bone lesions
- Other forms of thermal ablation use microwave, laser or high intensity focused ultrasound
- Cryoablation may be used to cause necrosis via rapid heating and thawing cyclically

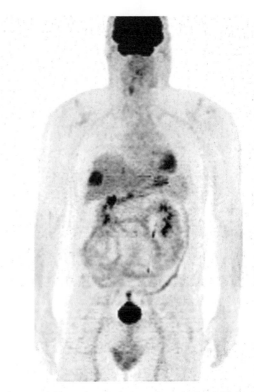

Figure 17.9 Coronal maximum intensity projection (MIP) image from the PET study.

Feasibility of resection depends upon the extent of disease, the condition of the underlying liver and the general health of the patient

- *Radiofrequency ablation* (Box 17.3) may be used alone, or in conjunction with either surgery or chemotherapy
- *Chemotherapy.* This may be used to reduce the extent of disease prior to surgery or alone, but is not usually curative in metastatic colorectal cancer.

The surgical team request that Mr Knight undergo a PET study. Why?

Positron emission tomography (PET) is the most sensitive imaging technique for detecting metastases in colorectal cancer. It enables detection of tumour within the liver not seen with CT, and in lymph nodes of normal size. PET is not used in surveillance because of the high cost, relatively limited availability and the significantly higher radiation dose.

The aim of the PET study is to ensure that hepatic resection will remove all detectable tumours; curative surgery is not usually attempted in the presence of extrahepatic disease within the abdomen but may be combined with thoracic resection in some cases.

What abnormality is shown here?

Within the right liver, there is a single large focus of FDG uptake which corresponds to the metastasis seen on the CT image (Fig. 17.9). The remaining areas of uptake (notably brain, heart, bowel and bladder) represent areas with a high metabolic activity and excretion of the FDG. There is no evidence of extrahepatic disease.

Mr Knight undergoes a right hepatectomy to resect the liver metastases. Four days after the operation, he becomes febrile, with an elevated white cell count and CRP.

What are the causes of a postoperative fever?

- Early (≤2 days):
  - haematoma, necrosis or tissue damage
  - chest infection
  - infection at operative site
  - blood transfusion
- 3–5 days:
  - wound infection

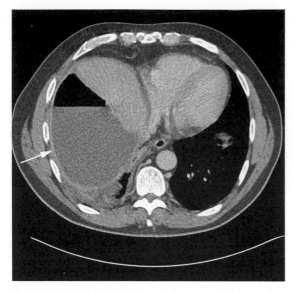

Figure 17.10 Axial CT image through the upper abdomen following administration of intravenous contrast medium.

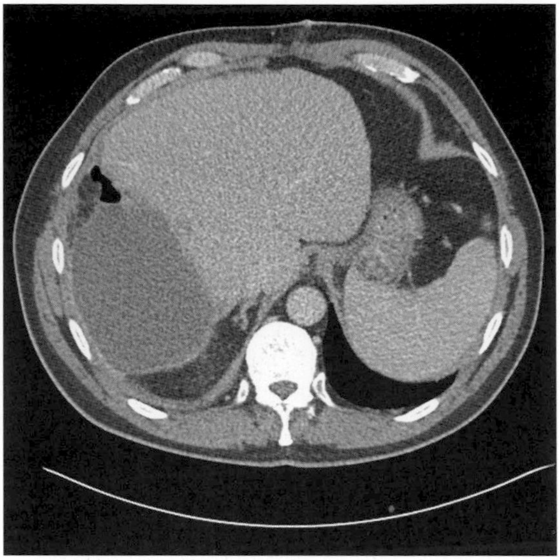

Figure 17.11 Axial CT image through the upper abdomen following administration of intravenous contrast medium.

- ○ chest infection
- ○ developing abdominal or pelvic abscess
- 5–7 days:
  - ○ anastamotic breakdown
  - ○ fistula formation
  - ○ venous thrombosis
- Late (>1 week):
  - ○ distant sepsis (e.g. subphrenic abscess)
  - ○ venous thrombosis

The wound is healing satisfactorily and the chest X-ray proves to be normal. Mr Knight is therefore referred for a CT of the abdomen and pelvis.

What do the images show?

In the surgical bed, following resection of the right liver, there is a large fluid collection with an air–fluid level seen anteriorly (Fig. 17.10, arrow & Fig. 17.11). This collection is abutting the cut-surface of the liver and is associated with a small reactive pleural effusion (seen posteriorly behind the diaphragm). The presence of air could be caused by either a gas-forming organism or, more likely, by reflux of air through the biliary tree from the duodenum.

How should this be managed?

- *Percutaneous drainage of the collection.* Otherwise there will be a reservoir of infection

- *Insertion of a biliary stent* – to give preferential biliary drainage in to the duodenum rather than via the cut-surface
- *Intravenous antibiotics* – to treat the infection, regimen to be guided by the sample from the drainage

A pigtail catheter was inserted in to the collection under ultrasound guidance and infected bile drained freely.

The endoscopic retrograde cholangiopancreatography (ERCP) images demonstrate the injection of contrast medium retrogradely in to the common bile duct. The ducts appear normal but the contrast medium spills out into the right subphrenic space (Fig. 17.12, arrow & Fig. 17.13). A plastic stent is placed in the lower end of the common bile duct to encourage the normal flow of bile in to the duodenum. The CT image following initial drainage and subsequent ERCP demonstrates (white) contrast medium from the ERCP in the collection (Fig. 17.14).

Following further drainage of the abscess and a course of antibiotics, Mr Knight was discharged home and follow-up imaging arranged. Initial imaging demonstrated no evidence of disease recurrence. However, further abnormalities were noted 18 months after the liver resection (2½ years after initial colorectal surgery).

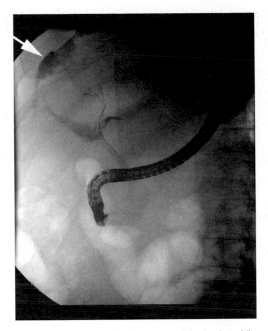

Figure 17.12 ERCP image showing contrast injection in to bile duct.

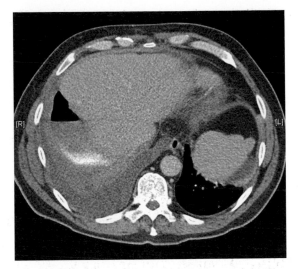

Figure 17.14 Axial CT image through the upper abdomen following ERCP.

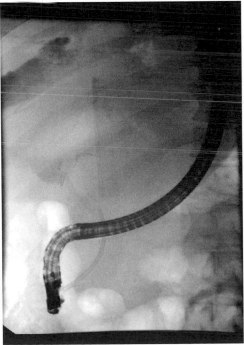

Figure 17.13 ERCP image demonstrating deployment of the biliary stent.

What do these images show?

Figure 17.15 demonstrates a further low attenuation metastatic deposit adjacent to the cut surface (Fig. 17.15, arrow). On the lower image at the level of the left portal vein (Fig. 17.16), one can appreciate how the residual left liver has hypertrophied over time when compared with the post-resection studies. The precise mechanism of what stimulates this hypertrophy of the liver (or indeed what stops it) is unclear at present. There are a number of simple cysts seen in the right kidney, of no clinical significance.

What therapeutic options are available at this stage?

The management options remain unchanged from the initial disease recurrence, but much will depend on the general health of the patient and the condition of the underlying liver. Patients who have received chemotherapy often have fatty infiltration and will require a greater residual volume of liver following the procedure. Leaving too little liver will result in liver failure.

Mr Knight underwent a further non-anatomical resection of the liver, i.e. the lesion was resected but not a whole liver segment. He made an uneventful recovery and remains well.

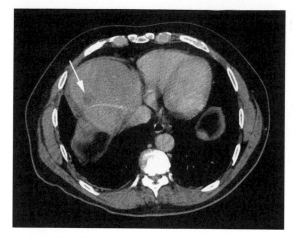

Figure 17.15 Axial CT image through the upper abdomen following administration of intravenous contrast medium.

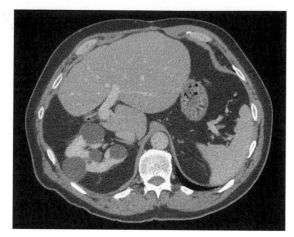

Figure 17.16 Axial CT image through the upper abdomen following administration of intravenous contrast medium.

CASE REVIEW

John Knight, a 67-year-old retired policeman, presented to his GP with rectal bleeding and visible haemorrhoids. His GP referred him to a colorectal surgeon for further management. She examined Mr Knight and found a craggy irregular mass on digital rectal examination. She proceeded to perform a rigid sigmoidoscopy in the outpatient clinic and took several biopsies of the rectal lesion.

Mr Knight was referred for an MRI of the rectum which demonstrated locally advanced disease involving the circumferential resection margin. Colonoscopy had to be abandoned because of the tortuous nature of the sigmoid colon, so Mr Knight underwent a CT colonography as part of his staging examination. A tiny polyp was found in the descending colon but no evidence of metastatic disease.

Mr Knight underwent a course of chemotherapy and radiotherapy, reducing the size of tumour significantly. At this point, surgical resection was performed with clear resection margins. Mr Knight commenced surveillance with a combination of colonoscopy and CT.

One year following the bowel surgery, a metastasis was found in the right liver at CT; this was confirmed to be solitary by a subsequent PET study. Surgical resection of this lesion was performed with a right hepatectomy. This was complicated by a biliary leak from the cut-surface which became infected. This was managed by percutaneous drainage, biliary stent insertion and a course of antibiotics.

Mr Knight resumed surveillance following his discharge. Unfortunately, 18 months later he developed a further metastasis at the cut-surface of the left liver. As Mr Knight was still in good health, with a normal underlying liver of adequate volume, he underwent a non-anatomical resection of the liver lesion which was uneventful. He remains disease-free at present.

KEY POINTS

- Never assume that rectal bleeding is caused by haemorrhoids
- Rectal examination is essential in all cases of rectal bleeding
- The diagnosis of cancer should be proven histologically, not just assumed from endoscopic appearances
- Staging of rectal cancer has three components: the mesorectum; the colon; the rest of the body
- The surgical procedure is a total mesorectal excision, either with an anastomosis (anterior resection) or, if the tumour is low, by removing the anus as well and leaving a colostomy (abdomino-perineal excision)
- If the resection margins are threatened or involved, preoperative chemo–radiotherapy should be performed
- If colonoscopy fails for any reason, CT colonography is the next best technique for evaluating the colon
- Postoperative surveillance of the colon and whole body should be performed to identify recurrence early
- The liver is the most common site of disease recurrence
- A number of options for treatment exist including surgery, thermal ablation and chemotherapy, depending on the clinical circumstances
- Imaging with PET is the most accurate means of detecting metastases, but screening is not feasible because of the cost and radiation dose
- Postoperative sepsis often needs a multidisciplinary approach to treat effectively

A 60-year-old woman with abdominal pain

Samantha Smith, a 60-year-old woman presents to her GP with a 2-week history of epigastric pain. She tells the GP that the pain 'comes and goes', and that it is unrelated to eating. She denies any recent weight loss, difficulty in swallowing or vomiting. She has not had any change in bowel habit, rectal bleeding or melaena. The GP examines her and finds a non-pulsatile epigastric mass which is a little tender.

What is the differential diagnosis of an epigastric mass?

- Stomach:
  - gastric malignancy
- Lymph nodes:
  - lymphoma
- Pancreas:
  - pancreatic cancer
  - pancreatic cyst
- Liver:
  - primary or secondary liver tumour
  - hepatic cyst
- Gallbladder:
  - empyema
  - mucocoele
- Aorta:
  - abdominal aortic aneurysm
- Transverse colon:
  - tumour
- Abdominal wall:
  - epigastric hernia

Radiology: Clinical Cases Uncovered. By A. S. Shaw, E. M. Godfrey, A. Singh and T. F. Massoud. Published 2009 by Blackwell Publishing. ISBN 978-1-4051-8474-8.

What blood tests would you request initially?

- Full blood count – to look for iron deficiency anaemia
- Liver function tests – to look for derangements of liver function that would suggest liver pathology or obstructed bile ducts

What else would you request in the first instance?

Mrs Smith has epigastric pain and a palpable mass. According to National Institute for Health and Clinical Excellence (NICE) guidelines (Box 18.1), she should be referred urgently for upper gastrointestinal endoscopy.

Mrs Smith asks you what an endoscopy involves. What do you tell her?

Before an upper gastrointestinal endoscopy she should fast: no solids for 6 hours and no liquids for 4 hours. She will be given topical local anaesthetic spray (which tastes unpleasant) in to the back of her throat. She may be sedated for the procedure. The person carrying out the endoscopy will then pass a flexible tube in to her mouth and down in to her stomach; the procedure lasts just a few minutes. If she requires intravenous sedation then she will not be able to drive herself home afterwards and should therefore take a friend or relative.

Should you start Mrs Smith on a proton pump inhibitor in case she has an ulcer?

No. Acid suppression with either a proton pump inhibitor (PPI) or an H_2-antagonist can mask and therefore delay diagnosis in patients with oesophageal or gastric cancer. If a patient is already taking a PPI then it should be stopped.

Box 18.1 NICE guidelines for upper gastrointestinal endoscopy

- Immediate (same day) specialist referral is indicated for patients presenting with dyspepsia together with significant acute gastrointestinal bleeding
- Urgent specialist referral or endoscopic investigation is indicated for patients of any age with dyspepsia when presenting with any of the following:
  - ○ chronic gastrointestinal bleeding
  - ○ progressive unintentional weight loss
  - ○ progressive difficulty swallowing
  - ○ persistent vomiting
  - ○ iron deficiency anaemia
  - ○ epigastric mass
  - ○ suspicious barium meal
- Review medications for possible causes of dyspepsia (e.g. calcium antagonists, nitrates, theophyllines, bisphosphonates, corticosteroids and non-steroidal anti-inflammatory drugs [NSAIDs]). In patients requiring referral, suspend NSAID use
- Consider the possibility of cardiac or biliary disease as part of the differential diagnosis

Mrs Smith attends for an upper gastrointestinal endoscopy. The findings are completely normal, as are the blood tests that were sent by the GP. The gastroenterologist performing the endoscopy subsequently examined Mrs Smith, confirming the previous finding of an epigastric mass; she requests an ultrasound of the abdomen.

What do the ultrasound images show?

The images in Figs 18.1–18.3 show the liver, gallbladder and common duct. The liver has a normal homogeneous echotexture and there are no mass lesions demonstrated. The gallbladder is free of calculi and the common bile duct is not dilated. The ultrasound report states that the liver, spleen and kidneys appear normal. The pancreas and aorta were not seen because of overlying bowel gas.

What would you do next?

In this case the cause of the epigastric mass has still not been discovered. A CT of the abdomen would be a reasonable next step to determine whether there is indeed an epigastric mass, and to characterize it.

What does the image show?

This axial CT image through the upper abdomen has been acquired following administration of intravenous

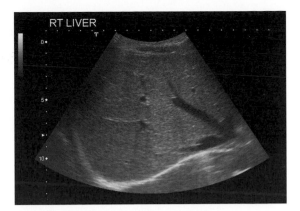
Figure 18.1 Image from the abdominal ultrasound.

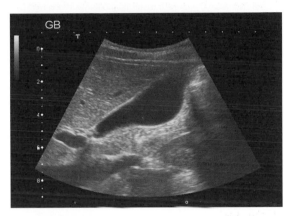
Figure 18.2 Image from the abdominal ultrasound.

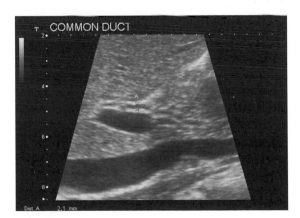
Figure 18.3 Image from the abdominal ultrasound.

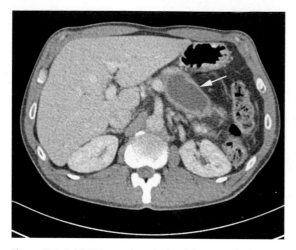

Figure 18.4 Axial CT image through the abdomen at the level of the pancreas.

contrast medium (Fig. 18.4). The stomach is seen anteriorly, the liver on the right and the kidneys posteriorly. On the left, the splenic flexure of the colon is seen. All of these structures have normal appearances. In the centre of the image there is a fluid-filled structure in the retroperitoneum, arising from and partially replacing the pancreas (Fig. 18.4, arrow).

What is the differential diagnosis of a cystic lesion arising of the pancreas?

- Inflammatory:
  - pseudocyst
- Neoplastic:
  - serous cystadenoma
  - mucinous cystic neoplasm
  - intraductal papillary mucinous neoplasm

There are a number of other, much rarer, cystic tumours as well as solid tumours that have undergone cystic degeneration that may be encountered.

Unlike the liver and kidneys, simple cysts with an epithelial lining are uncommon in the pancreas, but when they do occur they may be multiple. They are associated with the following conditions:

- Adult polycystic kidney disease
- von Hippel–Lindau syndrome
- Cystic fibrosis

The most frequently encountered cystic lesion in the pancreas is a pseudocyst. Pseudocysts evolve from acute peripancreatic fluid collections and occur in around 1 in 6 patients following an episode of acute pancreatitis.

They are most commonly found in the pararenal space or the lesser sac, but can track distally in to other locations such as the mediastinum. Pseudocysts consist of sterile pancreatic fluid, initially constrained by anatomical fascial planes, which become encapsulated by an inflammatory wall, a process that takes at least 4 weeks to occur. The typical CT features are of a fluid collection (<15 HU) with a smooth thin wall forming a round or ovoid configuration. Most pseudocysts, especially if under 6 cm, are asymptomatic and either resolve spontaneously or remain stable in size. Complications include haemorrhage and infection, as well as local pressure symptoms with larger cysts. In this case, it is unclear whether Mrs Smith has had an episode of pancreatitis or not.

With the increase in cross-sectional imaging worldwide, cystic tumours of the pancreas are increasingly detected; approximately 10% of cysts in the pancreas are malignant. Cross-sectional imaging of pancreatic cysts often gives a clue to the diagnosis and the likelihood of malignancy. Lesions that consist of multiple tiny cysts (microcystic) are almost always a serous cystadenoma. This is a benign tumour that requires no surgery. Conversely, multiple large cysts (macrocystic) throughout the lesion are seen with mucinous neoplasms. These have malignant potential and need surgical resection. Simple unilocular cysts are the most difficult to diagnose in many cases. Assuming that a pseudocyst has been excluded, mucinous tumours are the most likely aetiology. If the lesion measures <3 cm in diameter, they may be simply observed over a period of time as these are usually benign. When the diagnosis is in doubt, it is important to try to achieve a histological diagnosis wherever possible.

Although it is possible to perform CT-guided procedures on the pancreas, one often has to cross the liver and/or bowel to reach it. Consequently, endoscopic ultrasound has been developed to help diagnose and plan the management of patients with pancreatic lesions. The technical aspects of endoscopic ultrasound are described in Box 18.2; the applications and indications for endoluminal ultrasound are outlined in Box 18.3.

Mrs Smith was referred for endoscopic ultrasound and aspiration.

The images (Figs 18.5–18.8) show endoscopic aspiration, with complete collapse of the cyst. The cyst fluid was sent for analysis. It was found to contain abundant mucin,

Box 18.2 Endoscopic ultrasound

Endoscopic ultrasound is performed using a modified endoscope and has the same periprocedural requirements as endoscopy. In addition to the fibre-optic camera, an ultrasound probe is mounted on the distal end of the endoscope. This may be radial to give a 360° view or linear to give a longitudinal view of one segment. The small field of view involved enables higher resolution ultrasound images than would be possible with the ultrasound probe outside the patient. Using a linear ultrasound probe, the operator is also able to carry out aspiration of cysts, biopsy or fine-needle aspiration of lymph nodes or tumours

Box 18.3 Common indications for endoscopic ultrasound

Upper gastrointestinal
- Staging oesophageal cancer
- Diagnosis of and staging ampullary and pancreatic cancer
- Evaluation of the common bile duct for malignancy or calculi
- Lymph node sampling
- Pain relief (coeliac axis neurolysis)

Lower gastrointestinal
- Can be used for rectal cancer staging (particularly early stage)

Lung (endobronchial ultrasound)
- Diagnosis and staging of lung cancer
- Lymph node sampling

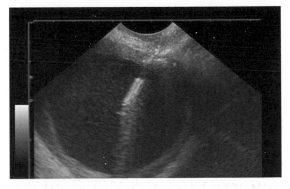

Figure 18.6 Endoscopic ultrasound image of the cyst with insertion of a needle.

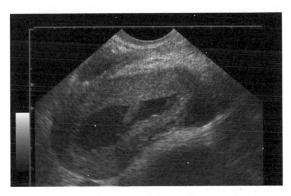

Figure 18.7 Endoscopic ultrasound image of the cyst during drainage.

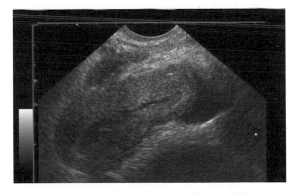

Figure 18.8 Endoscopic ultrasound image of the cyst following drainage showing complete collapse.

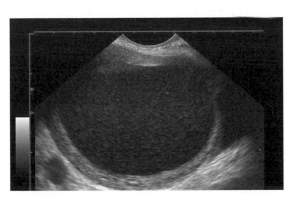

Figure 18.5 Endoscopic ultrasound image of the cyst within the pancreas.

indicative of a mucinous neoplasm (either a cystadenoma or cystadenocarcinoma).

In view of the potential malignancy, Mrs Smith was offered surgery in the form of a Whipple's procedure

(pancreaticoduodenectomy), to which she agreed. Postoperative histological examination confirmed the lesion to be mucinous cystadenoma, a benign tumour with malignant potential. Mrs Smith made an uneventful recovery.

CASE REVIEW

A 60-year-old woman presented with a 2-week history of episodic epigastric pain. On examination she was found to have an epigastric mass. She was referred for urgent endoscopy in accordance with established guidelines, but this was normal. Subsequently she was referred for an abdominal ultrasound, which was also normal.

However, in view of the clinical history, a CT examination of the abdomen was requested. This demonstrated a cystic pancreatic lesion with indeterminate features. An endoscopic ultrasound was performed to further evaluate the lesion and obtain a sample for cytology. Analysis of the cyst fluid suggested a mucinous neoplasm. This was confirmed histologically, after the patient underwent a Whipple's procedure.

KEY POINTS

- Patients with dyspepsia should be evaluated for symptoms and signs requiring urgent endoscopy
- A normal ultrasound does not rule out an epigastric mass; the pancreas is often obscured by bowel gas
- CT gives a good overview of the abdomen, enabling visualization of both the solid organs and the bowel
- Pancreatic lesions may often be characterized by their CT appearances

- Endoscopic ultrasound enables high resolution diagnostic images to be taken and aspiration or biopsy of a lesion
- Small unilocular cysts are usually benign
- Mucinous tumours require surgical resection because of their malignant potential

Case 19 A 34-year-old man with microscopic haematuria

Jonathan Brown, a 34-year-old pilot, attended a health screening clinic for a routine medical examination as part of a pre-employment screening check. Mr Brown, a married father of three children, felt well and had no history of any medical problems at all. He is a lifelong non-smoker and drinks very little alcohol. Clinical examination is entirely normal, but a urine dipstick test revealed there to be a trace of blood. There was no evidence of protein or glucose.

What are the potential causes of microscopic haematuria in this patient?

There are numerous potential causes for haematuria, and many potential sites. Hence, one needs to adopt a systematic approach:

- Renal:
  - glomerular disease
  - interstitial disease (e.g. infection, papillary necrosis)
  - cystic disease
  - stone disease
  - trauma
  - malignancy
- Ureter:
  - stone disease
  - malignancy
- Bladder:
  - stone disease
  - infection
  - malignancy
- Prostate:
  - prostatitis
  - malignancy
- Urethra:
  - urethritis
  - trauma

Radiology: Clinical Cases Uncovered. By A. S. Shaw, E. M. Godfrey, A. Singh and T. F. Massoud. Published 2009 by Blackwell Publishing. ISBN 978-1-4051-8474-8.

In such a young patient, who is a non-smoker, the risk of malignancy is very low. Recent trauma can also be excluded very easily by asking the patient about this specifically.

What investigations would you request at this stage?

- Urine:
  - microscopy and culture – to confirm the presence of red blood cells and look for evidence of renal disease or infection
- Blood:
  - urea and electrolytes – to check renal function
- Radiology:
  - ultrasound of the renal tract
  - abdominal X-ray

What do these images show?

The ultrasound of the left kidney is normal (Figs 19.1 & 19.2). In the right kidney, there is a focal area of increased echogenicity at the lower pole with an acoustic shadow behind it (Fig. 19.3, arrow & Fig. 19.4). The plain film confirms the presence of a right renal calculus (Fig. 19.5).

The urine microscopy confirms the presence of red blood cells in the urine, but there are no other cells and no casts. Urine culture was negative and renal function was normal. Therefore Mr Brown was referred to a urologist for follow-up of his renal calculi. As Mr Brown is asymptomatic, it was decided to manage the renal calculi conservatively and to monitor the calculi.

What do renal calculi consist of?

There are several different types of renal calculi, each of which has a different underlying aetiology. These are listed in Box 19.1.

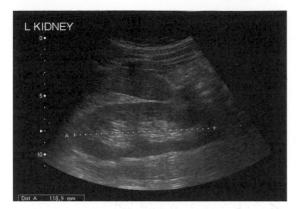

Figure 19.1 Longitudinal ultrasound image of the left kidney.

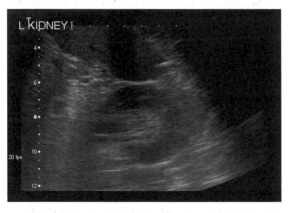

Figure 19.2 Transverse ultrasound image of the left kidney.

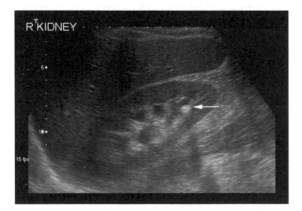

Figure 19.3 Longitudinal ultrasound image of the right kidney.

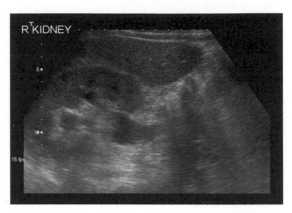

Figure 19.4 Transverse ultrasound image of the right kidney.

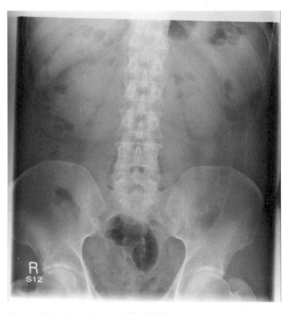

Figure 19.5 Plain abdominal film (KUB).

Box 19.1 Composition of renal calculi

Calcium oxalate/phosphate/apatite (75%)

- Often associated with metabolic disorders resulting in hypercalciuria or hyperoxaluria
- Hypercalciuria – hyperparathyroidism, neoplastic disease, Cushing's syndrome, hyperthyroidism, demineralization secondary to immobilization, hypervitaminosis D, sarcoidosis
- Hyperoxaluria – oxalosis, inflammatory bowel disease (especially Crohn's disease), pyridoxine (vitamin B_6) deficiency
- In 25% of cases there is no underlying metabolic disorder

Struvate (15%)

- Urinary tract infections, in particular with urea-splitting organisms such as *Proteus mirabilis*
- Urinary stasis

Urate (6%)

- Hyperuricaemia – uricosuria, usually secondary to treatment for gout (uricosuric agents), or for myeloproliferative disorders (chemotherapeutic agents)
- 50% are idiopathic

Cystine (2%)

- secondary to hypercystinuria, an autosomal recessive disorder resulting in abnormal renal tubular reabsorption of cystine

Xanthine

- Hyperxanthinuria – deficiency of xanthine oxidase, necessary for the conversion of xanthine to uric acid in purine catabolism

Drug associated

- Indinavir (antiretroviral agent)
- Magnesium silicate (excessive use of some antacids)
- Sulfs-drugs (e.g. sulfasalazine)

What proportion of renal calculi can be seen on the plain film?

Most calculi can be detected on plain X-rays; however, it is often difficult to localize them to the ureters, and differentiation from other calcification severely limits the sensitivity of plain radiography for ureteral stones. Approximately 4% of renal calculi (predominantly those composed of urate and xanthine) are radiolucent on plain X-rays.

How should Mr Brown be followed up radiologically?

Asymptomatic renal calculi may be followed either by serial plain films or by CT. The former results in a lower radiation dose to the patient but the latter gives a more precise evaluation of the exact size and number of calculi and their distribution. In a young patient such as Mr Brown, one would be very keen to minimize radiation exposure. As the calculi were visible on the plain film, this is preferable in this case.

Why does the urologist not follow Mr Brown with ultrasound?

Ultrasound has a very low sensitivity for stone detection, identifying only around one-quarter of calculi. Only calculi greater than 5 mm in size can be reliably identified in the pelvicalyceal system. The smaller the stone, the less likely it is to cast an acoustic shadow. Ureteric stones are very poorly visualized unless they are within the proximal ureter or at the vesico-ureteric junction. Consequently, it is of limited value in this situation.

> Mr Brown declines any therapy as he feels well, and so was followed in the outpatient department for several years by the urological team without any change in the appearances of the abdominal film and without any further symptoms.
>
> Six years later, he presented late at night to the accident and emergency department with severe right-sided abdominal pain. It had begun earlier in the day and had become progressively worse. On questioning, he described the pain as 'unbearable' and had no relief from simple analgesia. On examination, Mr Brown was found to be pale, sweating and clutching his right side. You assess Mr Brown:
>
> | | |
> |---|---|
> | Airway | Patent; patient talking in full sentences |
> | Breathing | Respiratory rate 20 breaths/minute |
> | | Oxygen saturation 98% breathing room air |
> | Circulation | Pulse 105 beats/minute, regular |
> | | Blood pressure 140/75 mmHg |
> | Disposition | In obvious severe pain |

What should you do in the first instance?

- Analgesia
- Anti-emetics (if required)

As Mr Brown is in severe pain, one should rapidly administer analgesia to help with the pain. This will enable you to obtain a full clinical history and perform an examination; analgesia will not mask significant clinical signs.

What are the key points to cover in the clinical history?

- Pain:
  - site and radiation
  - onset and progression
  - aggravating and/or alleviating factors
  - severity
- Previous episodes
- Associated symptoms:
  - urinary
  - bowel
- Past medical history

> His pain partially relieved, Mr Brown was able to describe the pain as mostly dull but occasionally sharp, coming in 'waves' but never going away completely. The pain seems to be centred on the right flank, occasionally radiating down to his right groin. He scores the pain as '10/10', being the worst pain he has ever experienced and having never occurred before. He has vomited once, shortly after the pain began. He has not had any food or fluids since, has not opened his bowels and passed very little urine.
>
> On examination, although apyrexial, he was pale and sweaty, his obvious discomfort meaning that he could not lie still for long. His abdomen was soft and non-tender with no masses. Digital rectal examination was normal. Urinalysis demonstrated 2+ blood, but was otherwise normal.

What is the most likely diagnosis?

The clinical signs and symptoms all point to right-sided renal colic. Given the clinical history and in the absence of a fever, further investigations should be directed towards proving this diagnosis and looking for the complications of renal tract calculi.

You request a plain radiograph (KUB) but the radiographer refuses. Why?

Mr Brown's symptoms suggest that there is a calculus within the renal tract that is causing symptomatic obstruction or is passing down the ureter. Although the plain film (kidney, ureter and bladder [KUB]) will demonstrate the renal calculi, it is much harder to identify ureteric calculi (and distinguish them from calcified lymph nodes or phleboliths), particularly when positioned in the pelvis. Furthermore, the plain film will not demonstrate the complications of renal calculi (principally, renal tract obstruction). Hence, the plain film has

---

> **Box 19.2 Intravenous urography**
>
> - Used in the evaluation of renal disease for several decades
> - Abdominal radiograph is acquired
> - Intravenous contrast medium is injected by hand
> - Further radiographs are acquired at different time intervals
> - Demonstrates the passage of contrast medium through the renal tract during excretion
> - Non-functioning kidneys may not be seen
> - Obstructed kidneys may take many hours to opacify
> - Now almost completely replaced by CT imaging

little or no value in the setting of acute renal colic, and as such the radiographer is right to say that the study (and radiation exposure) is not justified in the emergency situation.

However, X-rays may be useful as a baseline for the radiologist or urologist for further follow-up studies and sometimes are useful to monitor passage of a confirmed radio-opaque stone.

What radiological investigation should be requested?

A CT of the abdomen and pelvis is the most appropriate investigation. Unenhanced CT has revolutionized the imaging of renal stone disease, particularly in the acute setting, with the intravenous urogram (IVU) (Box 19.2) now almost obsolete. Almost all (99%) calculi are radio-opaque on CT and are identified as geometric or oval high attenuation foci with an attenuation of at least 150 Hounsfield units (HU). This also allows easy differentiation of calculi from other renal tract lesions such as tumours and haematomas which are usually less than 50 HU. When there is difficulty determining whether a focus of calcification is in the ureter or outside it, intravenous contrast medium may be given to opacify the ureters.

The power of CT is further enhanced by the ability to reconstruct the images in multiple planes. Additionally, CT allows the identification of other differential diagnoses of abdominal pain where a ureteric calculus is not the cause.

Is there any place for magnetic resonance imaging?

Magnetic resonance urography avoids ionizing radiation but is less sensitive, more expensive and takes longer to

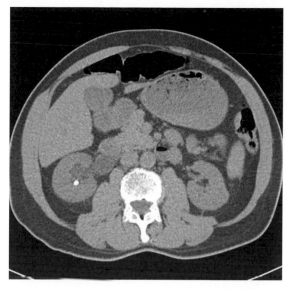

Figure 19.6 Axial unenhanced CT image through the renal hila.

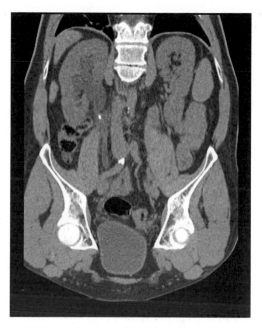

Figure 19.8 Coronal reconstruction of the unenhanced CT study.

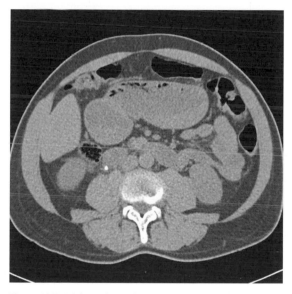

Figure 19.7 Axial unenhanced image at the level of the proximal ureters.

Box 19.3 **Common sites of calculus impaction**

- In the kidney:
  - minor and major calyx system
  - pelvi-ureteric junction
- In the ureter:
  - pelvic brim – where the ureter arches over the iliac vessels
  - vesico ureteric junction – the most narrow part of the normal urinary tract
- In the bladder:
  - usually do not originate from the upper tracts and instead form *in situ*

  Calculi originating from the upper tracts found in the bladder are likely to pass easily through the urethra

perform. Consequently, it is reserved for a few specific indications, notably in the evaluation of pregnant women.

What does this unenhanced CT of the kidney, ureter and bladder show?

Figure 19.6 demonstrates dilatation of the right-sided renal collecting system with a calculus *in situ*. Figure 19.7 demonstrates a further calcific density within the right ureter. The coronal reformatted image (Fig. 19.8) elegantly demonstrates how the calculus is resulting in hydronephrosis of the right kidney.

What are the typical sites where renal calculi cause obstruction?

The calculi typically obstruct at points of relative narrowing within the renal tract, listed in Box 19.3.

Mr Brown was referred to the urology team for further management.

What management options are available to the urological team?

There are a number of approaches available for the management of renal tract calculi:

• *Extracorporeal shock wave lithotripsy* (ESWL). High intensity sound waves are used to shatter large renal calculi so that they pass of their own accord

• *Percutaneous nephrolithotomy* (PCNL). A nephrostomy is performed and the track dilated until an endoscope can be passed through it. The calculi are then removed individually from the kidney

• *Open surgery* to either remove calculi or perform a nephrectomy. As a 'rule of thumb', a nephrectomy may be considered if the contribution of the affected kidney to total renal function is <10%, and any associated obstruction or sepsis has been treated

• *Cystoscopy and/or ureteroscopy and stone removal.* Using a retrograde approach, the calculi are removed or crushed endoscopically

• *Expectant management*:
  ○ 80% of calculi 4 mm in diameter will pass spontaneously
  ○ 20% of calculi 5 mm in diameter will pass spontaneously

Mr Brown underwent a retrograde ureteroscopy to remove the obstructing calculus and made an uneventful recovery.

CASE REVIEW

Jonathan Brown, a 34-year-old pilot, attended a pre-employment health check and was found to have microscopic haematuria with normal renal function. Investigation with a plain abdominal radiograph and renal ultrasound revealed the presence of calculi. As he was asymptomatic, Mr Brown declined any treatment and was followed up in the outpatient department by the urological team.

Six years later, Mr Brown presented to his local accident and emergency department with severe right-sided colicky abdominal pain. An unenhanced CT revealed a calculus obstructing the right ureter. The urologists were informed and proceeded to remove the calculus using a ureteroscope. Mr Brown made an uneventful recovery.

KEY POINTS

• The radiological investigation of renal disease depends on the presenting complaint

• Microscopic haematuria should be investigated with an ultrasound and abdominal X-ray

• Most calculi can be detected on plain radiographs but often add little to the emergent clinical impression

• Ultrasound has a relatively low sensitivity for renal calculus detection but is useful to rule out potential complications of urinary tract calculi, in particular, hydronephrosis

• IVU is rarely performed nowadays, but can give anatomical and functional information relating to the renal tract

• Almost all calculi are detectable using unenhanced CT, which is currently the gold standard for detecting renal tract calculi

• CT allows the radiologist to identify complications of stone disease (e.g. obstruction)

• CT imaging also allows the identification of other causes of abdominal pain where a ureteric calculus is not present

• MRI may be useful in specific situations (e.g. in pregnancy)

• Prompt and aggressive management of complications of obstructing calculi, such as hydronephrosis and pyelonephritis, is paramount

• Management involves close collaboration between both the urologist and radiologist

Case 20 # A 53-year-old man with frank haematuria

Joshua Green, a 53-year-old builder, presents to his GP complaining of having passed what he thinks is blood in his urine for the past 2 days. He had never visited his doctor before and had no other medical complaints; hence he was rather alarmed at the sight of pink urine.

What key features would you ask about in the clinical history?

The differential diagnosis for patients with haematuria is wide, as discussed in Case 19. In order to try and narrow down the possibilities, there are a few key questions:
• Is there any associated pain?
  ○ due to stones or blood clots
• Are there any blood clots? If so, what shape are they?
  ○ worm-like suggests ureteric
  ○ different shapes suggests prostate or urethra
• Has Mr Green passed any stones?
• Has there been any trauma?
• Is there any reason to suspect infection?
  ○ unprotected sexual intercourse?
• Is the blood at the start of the urine flow or throughout?
  ○ urethral causes may see blood just at the start

Mr Green reports that he has had some mild left-sided pain, but this had resolved with paracetamol. He could not think of any significant trauma, had not passed any stones or blood clots to his knowledge and had not had sexual intercourse with anyone except his wife of 24 years. He thought that the blood was present throughout urination.

What test should you perform in clinic?

It is worth testing a urine sample for the presence of blood even if it looks discolored as certain foods can

Radiology: Clinical Cases Uncovered. By A. S. Shaw, E. M. Godfrey, A. Singh and T. F. Massoud. Published 2009 by Blackwell Publishing. ISBN 978-1-4051-8474-8.

cause urine discoloration. A further sample should be sent for urine microscopy and culture to look for infection.

Urinalysis indicates that there is indeed blood in Mr Green's urine. He asks you whether or not you think he has cancer.

What are the risk factors for developing a urothelial tumour?

In the Western population there are three main risk factors:

1 Smoking
2 Age >40 years
3 Exposure to aromatic amines, particularly petrochemical, plastics, textiles and printing industries

In tropical countries, chronic infection with *Schistosoma haematobium* is the major aetiological factor. Analgesic abuse is associated with developing urothelial tumours, but this is much less common. At times, various foods have been linked with bladder tumours but these have subsequently been disproved.

Mr Green smoked 20 cigarettes a day from the age of 15 until he was 33 years old but has not smoked since. He tells you that he has never worked as anything other than a builder.

How might you investigate the cause of Mr Green's haematuria?

Most centres will stratify the investigation of patients with frank haematuria according to the risk that they have an underlying tumour. Patients with one or more of the above risk factors may be considered 'high-risk', while non-smokers under 40 years of age are considered to be 'low-risk'. For patients with frank haematuria at high risk, a combination of CT urography (Box 20.1) and flexible cystoscopy is advocated, whereas for those

> **Box 20.1 CT urography**
>
> CT urography is a study optimized for the evaluation of the kidneys, ureters and bladder. As such, it is performed in a different manner from a standard CT of the abdomen and pelvis. Initially, an unenhanced study is peformed to look for renal tract calculi. Following administration of intravenous contrast medium, several discrete phases are seen on renal imaging:
> - Corticomedullary phase
> - Nephrographic phase
> - Excretory phase
>
> In order to avoid the radiation dose that would be associated with four CT studies, the dose of intravenous contrast medium is divided and given at predetermined intervals. Then, a single phase of imaging is performed such that the first bolus of contrast medium is in the excretory phase, and later bolus(es) are in the nephrographic +/– corticomedullary phase according to local protocols.
>
> Images are often reconstructed in the coronal or even curved planes to give an image resembling an intravenous urogram. This is the most sensitive radiological technique for evaluating the renal tract.

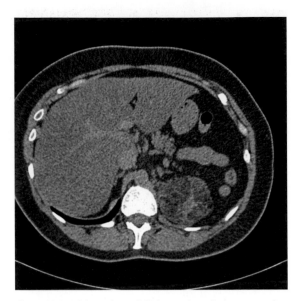

Figure 20.1 Axial unenhanced CT image through the upper pole of the left kidney.

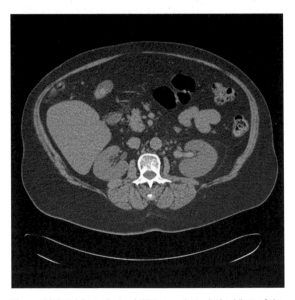

Figure 20.2 Axial unenhanced CT image through the hilum of the left kidney.

patients considered to be at low risk, many choose to avoid the radiation associated with CT and combine a renal ultrasound with flexible cystoscopy. This latter approach is far less sensitive for tumour detection.

Joshua was referred to the 'one-stop' haematuria clinic at his local hospital. In view of his risk factors (age and smoking), he underwent CT urography followed by flexible cystoscopy. Images from the CT urography study are shown in Figs 20.1 and 20.2.

What do these images show?

Figure 20.1 demonstrates a mass arising from the upper pole of the left kidney. The lesion appears rather heterogeneous but, crucially, contains several areas of very low attenuation compared with that of the subcutaneous fat. Therefore, one can deduce from this single image that this lesion represents an angiomyolipoma (AML; Box 20.2). In Fig. 20.2, compare the density of the left and right ureters on these unenhanced images. The left side is denser and this suggests that there is high density material, probably blood, within the left ureter. However, there is no evidence of renal obstruction. The combina-

tion of these images strongly suggests that the AML is, or has recently been, bleeding.

The radiographer asks 'Is there any value in the second stage of the study?'

The purpose of the investigation is twofold: to look for a cause of bleeding and to exclude a urothelial tumour. The

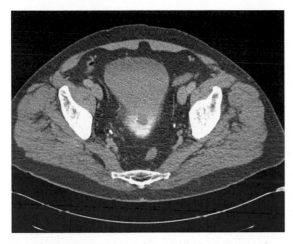

Figure 20.3 Axial CT image through the bladder following intravenous contrast medium.

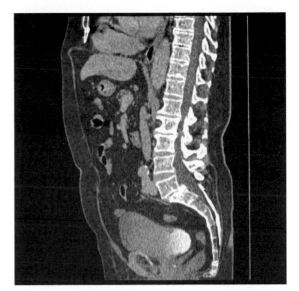

Figure 20.4 Midline sagittal reconstruction CT image following intravenous contrast medium.

Box 20.2 Renal angiomyolipoma

As the name suggests, this is a benign neoplasm composed of vascular smooth muscle and fatty elements, with the demonstration of the latter being virtually pathognomonic. It is worth noting that fat may be present only in microscopic amounts in up to 5% of cases. Other key features are:

- 4 female: 1 male
- Present in up to 3% of the population
- 80% sporadic; 20% associated with tuberous sclerosis
- Of sporadic cases, 40% are symptomatic
- Symptoms are more common in larger tumours (>4 cm)
- Rupture may cause life-threatening haemorrhage
- Treatment options include embolization or resection

Box 20.3 Transitional cell carcinoma of the bladder

- Fourth most common tumour in men; tenth most common in women
- Multicentricity and metachronous tumours are common
- Represents >90% of bladder tumours:
  - ≤5% are squamous cell carcinoma
  - 2% are adenocarcinoma
- Three times more common in men
- Risk factors:
  - age >40 years
  - smoking
  - aromatic amine exposure
  - analgesic abuse
  - *Schistosoma haematobium* infection

---

two aims should be considered independently and the study only considered to be complete when a full evaluation of the renal tract has been made.

What do these images show?

Figures 20.3 and 20.4 elegantly demonstrate the presence of a filling defect within the superior aspect of the bladder. This does not contain any calcification and is not dependent within the bladder. The features are strongly suggestive of a bladder tumour.

Later the same morning, Joshua underwent a flexible cystoscopy which confirmed the bladder tumour. A biopsy was taken from the tumour which was subsequently

reported as a high grade transitional cell carcinoma (Box 20.3). Two weeks later, surgical resection of the tumour was performed and this was reported to be T2 disease by the histopathologist (Box 20.4).

How should this be treated?

Early stage disease (CIS, Ta, T1) that is not invading muscle may be treated by a combination of local resection and bacille Calmette–Guérin (BCG) immunotherapy. However, those patients with proven muscle-invasive disease, as in this case, should undergo a cystectomy.

> **Box 20.4** **Bladder tumour staging**
>
> The TNM staging system for bladder cancer is:
> | | |
> |---|---|
> | CIS | Carcinoma *in situ*, high grade dysplasia, confined to the epithelium |
> | Ta | Papillary tumour confined to the epithelium |
> | T1 | Tumour invasion in to the lamina propria |
> | T2 | Tumour invasion in to the muscularis propria |
> | T3 | Tumour involvement of the periveiseal fat |
> | T4 | Tumour involvement of adjacent organs such as prostate, rectum or pelvic sidewall |
> | N+ | Presence of lymph node metastasis |
> | M+ | Presence of distant metastasis |

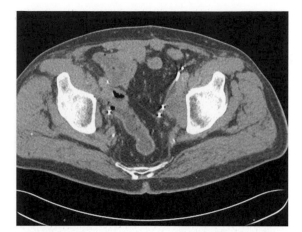

Figure 20.5 Axial CT image through the pelvis following intravenous contrast medium.

Joshua underwent a radiological embolization of the left renal AML and then proceeded to a radical cystectomy for his bladder tumour. This involves excision of the bladder, prostate and some of the pelvic lymph nodes. Following the procedure, Joshua complained of groin pain on the left side which was thought to be 'post-surgical'. One month following surgery, the discomfort persisted and he was referred for a CT study.

What does this image show?

In Fig. 20.5 surgical clips can be seen within the pelvis following the recent surgery, the high density metal causing some minor artefacts. Between the left side of the bony pelvis and the surgical clips is an area of abnormal soft tissue.

What could this represent?

This could be one of two things:

1 Tumour recurrence
2 Postoperative haematoma

In view of the recent surgery and postoperative symptoms, it was felt more likely that this represented a postoperative haematoma. Joshua's symptoms subsequently subsided. However, to confirm that this was a haematoma, a further study was requested 2 months later.

What does this image show?

In Fig. 20.6 the soft tissue mass abutting the left pelvic sidewall has increased in size compared with the previous study. This confirms that the mass is tumour rather than haematoma as previously suspected.

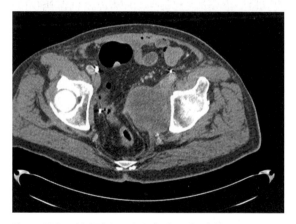

Figure 20.6 Axial CT image through the pelvis following intravenous contrast medium.

Joshua was referred for chemotherapy and had a complete response, the enlarged lymph nodes resolving entirely. He remained on regular surveillance with CT without any concern for the next 15 months, but then developed further haematuria. Further CT urography was attempted but the images were suboptimal because of dilatation of the upper renal tracts following radical cystectomy.

Why might the upper tracts be dilated?

Following a radical cystectomy, a neo-bladder is created from bowel to which the ureters are anastamosed. These anastamoses do not have the same anti-reflux configuration as the normal vesico-ureteric junction and hence reflux is considered 'normal'. Conversely, strictures may form as with any other anastomosis and thus dilatation may indicate obstruction.

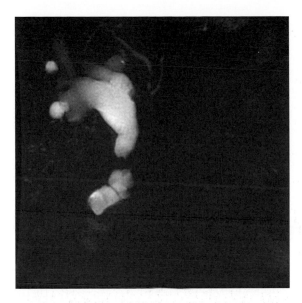

Figure 20.7 Coronal T2-weighted image of the right ureter from a magnetic resonance urography study.

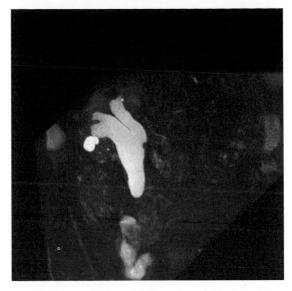

Figure 20.8 Coronal oblique T2-weighted image of the right ureter from a magnetic resonance urography study.

What other options are available?

The dilated ureters reduce the sensitivity of any investigation that requires instillation of contrast medium as they will cause dilution. Magnetic resonance urography images the fluid in the collecting system without contrast medium. Alternatively, ureteroscopy could be performed.

What do these images show?

In Figs 20.7 and 20.8 the right ureter and renal pelvis are markedly dilated. On the medial wall of the upper ureter is a small round area which returns a low signal. This appears to be arising from the wall of the ureter and is almost certainly tumour recurrence.

Joshua underwent a retrograde ureteroscopy with biopsy which confirmed the findings of the MRI study. He subsequently underwent a right nephro-ureterectomy for the tumour recurrence and remains well under regular surveillance.

CASE REVIEW

Joshua Green, a 53-year-old builder, presented with a 2-day history of passing frank blood in his urine and mild left-sided discomfort relieved by simple analgesia. He had no risk factors for infection and had not been involved in any accidents to suggest renal tract trauma. Having confirmed that there was indeed blood in his urine, he was referred to the local haematuria clinic for further investigation.

From the referral, the risk of there being an underlying malignancy was assessed in order to determine the most appropriate investigations. Joshua's age (>40 years) and smoking history meant that he was considered to be at high risk. Therefore he underwent CT urography and flexible cystoscopy.

The unenhanced CT study showed a large left-sided renal AML with blood in the left ureter indicating either active or recent bleeding. Following administration of intravenous contrast medium, a small tumour could be seen arising from the superior wall of the bladder. At cystoscopy, this tumour was biopsied and confirmed to be a high grade transitional cell carcinoma. Excision of the tumour revealed it to be invading the muscle (stage T2)

Continued

and hence Joshua subsequently underwent a radical cystectomy.

Following the procedure, Joshua complained of a persistent ache in his groin. A CT study performed 1 month after the operation identified a soft tissue mass at the left pelvic sidewall. In view of the symptoms, size and relationship to surgery this was thought most likely to represent a haematoma. However, the imaging was repeated after a short interval and the mass found to be significantly larger.

Joshua was referred for chemotherapy and underwent a complete response to chemotherapy. Over a year passed before Joshua developed further haematuria and underwent an MRI study of the ureters. This demonstrated a focal mass arising from the medial wall of a dilated right ureter and he had further surgery to remove the right kidney and ureter. This went smoothly and he remains well.

KEY POINTS

- There are many causes for frank haematuria
- Clinical history may exclude some causes, e.g. trauma
- Urine should be analysed for blood and infection
- Investigations should be tailored to balance the risk from the investigations with the risk of an underlying malignancy
- Ultrasound is preferred in low-risk patients
- CT urography is the optimal imaging study for high-risk patients or those with persistent haematuria
- Flexible cystoscopy is used to evaluate the bladder
- Early disease may be treated with local resection and immunotherapy
- Advanced disease requires radical cystectomy
- Surveillance should be carried out to look for metachronous urothelial tumours together with nodal or metastatic spread

A 69-year-old woman with post-menopausal bleeding

Jane Howell, a 69-year-old woman, presents to her GP with a 2-week history of vaginal bleeding. The key features of her clinical history are given in Box 21.1. The GP performs abdominal and vaginal examinations which are both normal.

What is the differential diagnosis for post-menopausal bleeding?

- Endometrial atrophy
- Endometrial hyperplasia
- Endometrial polyp
- Submucosal fibroid
- Endometrial carcinoma

Does Mrs Howell have any risk factors for endometrial cancer?

Most of the risk factors for endometrial cancer relate to the patient's exposure to unopposed oestrogen. Mrs Howell is taking tamoxifen following her previous breast cancer. This is a selective oestrogen receptor modulator, which means that it acts as a competitive antagonist in breast tissue (therefore reducing the risk of breast cancer recurrence), but as a partial agonist in endometrial tissue. It is associated with a threefold increase in the risk of developing endometrial cancer. Furthermore, she is nulliparous, which increases the risk of endometrial cancer (as well as breast cancer).

Rather unusually, smoking appears to be relatively protective against developing endometrial cancer, so as a non-smoker she is at increased risk. However, the benefit is small and far outweighed by the increased risk of developing many other cancers, ischaemic heart disease, chronic lung disease and a host of other conditions. Box 21.2 lists the risk factors for endometrial cancer.

Radiology: Clinical Cases Uncovered. By A. S. Shaw, E. M. Godfrey, A. Singh and T. F. Massoud. Published 2009 by Blackwell Publishing. ISBN 978-1-4051-8474-8.

What should the GP do next?

Although most patients with post-menopausal bleeding will have a benign cause (such as endometrial atrophy), the possibility of endometrial cancer is a concern and should be actively excluded. The patient should be referred to a gynaecologist, ideally offering a 'one-stop' clinic for clinical and radiological assessment.

The GP takes blood samples and refers Mrs Howell to a one-stop clinic for post-menopausal bleeding.

What investigations are required?

- Full blood count – to check for anaemia or thrombocytopenia
- Clotting – to look for a bleeding diathesis
- Pelvic ultrasound – transabdominal/transvaginal (Box 21.3)

Mrs Howell attends the one-stop clinic and undergoes transabdominal and transvaginal ultrasounds.

How have these images been acquired?

Figures 21.1 and 21.2 show the ultrasound probe at the top of the image and are transabdominal. In contrast, Figs 21.3 and 21.4 are transvaginal – the probe is at the bottom of the image, with the ultrasound beam angled upwards.

What do the images show?

The transabdominal ultrasound images show a complex cystic structure. The smaller of the two cystic parts measures approximately 3 cm and is anechoic (i.e. appears black). The larger measures approximately 10 cm in diameter and has internal echoes (i.e. appears grey). A structure as large as this would be difficult to fully delineate via the transvaginal approach.

The transvaginal ultrasound images show the uterus in axial and sagittal planes. The endometrium has been

---

Box 21.1 Clinical history

Presenting complaint. Vaginal bleeding for 2 weeks
History of presenting complaint. No precipitating
factors
    Menarche aged 12 years
    Menopause aged 51 years
Previous medical history. Breast cancer aged 67 years.
This was treated with wide local excision and sentinel
node biopsy
Drug history. Tamoxifen 20 mg o.d.
Family history. Nil
Social history. Lives with husband who is well
    She is not sexually active
    Never pregnant
    Non-smoker

Box 21.2 Risk factors for endometrial cancer

Risk factors
- Early menarche
- Late menopause
- Nulliparity
- Obesity
- Oestrogen-only hormone replacement therapy
- Tamoxifen
- Oestrogen-secreting ovarian tumours such as granulosa
  cell tumours
- Endometrial hyperplasia

Protective factors
- Smoking
- Oral contraceptive pill

Box 21.3 Transvaginal ultrasound

- Transvaginal ultrasound is complementary to 'standard'
  transabdominal ultrasound in imaging the female pelvis.
  Both have strengths and weaknesses and are therefore
  used in combination in adult women
- Transabdominal ultrasound is able to visualize to a
  greater depth, because the probe frequency is lower
  than those used for transvaginal ultrasound. This makes
  it ideal for assessing large pelvic masses. A full bladder
  is necessary to displace loops of bowel that would
  otherwise obscure the pelvic organs. This part of the
  examination is therefore usually carried out first
- Transvaginal ultrasound probes tend to have a higher
  frequency. This limits their potential depth, but increases
  image resolution. This makes transvaginal ultrasound
  ideal for the visualization of small structures such as the
  endometrium and ovaries. An empty bladder is
  necessary for patient comfort
- When referring young patients for pelvic ultrasound, it is
  important to realize that transvaginal approach is not
  considered appropriate in those patients who have not
  begun sexual activity

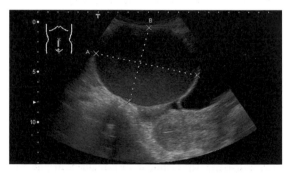

Figure 21.1 Transabdominal image from the pelvic ultrasound
examination.

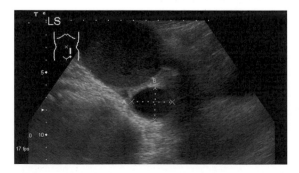

Figure 21.2 Transabdominal image from the pelvic ultrasound
examination.

---

measured and is 15 mm. This is abnormally thickened for
a post-menopausal woman (the maximum allowable is
5 mm).

What should happen next?

There are two issues here: an abnormally thickened
endometrium and a complex cystic pelvic mass.

The thickened endometrium should be evaluated histologically. There are a variety of possible approaches,
but a pipelle biopsy would be a reasonable approach. A
suction tube is introduced in to the uterus via a speculum
and samples are taken randomly. This procedure is performed on an outpatient basis and is therefore ideal in
the setting of a one-stop clinic. Providing a sufficient

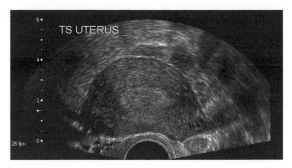

Figure 21.3 Transvaginal image from the pelvic ultrasound examination.

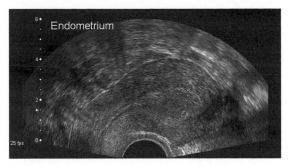
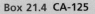

Figure 21.4 Transvaginal image from the pelvic ultrasound examination.

> **Box 21.4 CA-125**
>
> - CA-125 (cancer antigen-125) is a glycoprotein tumour marker
> - A raised level is associated with ovarian cancer, but it is neither highly sensitive nor specific
> - It may also be elevated in a variety of other cancers such as endometrial, lung, breast and colorectal
> - CA-125 may be raised in a number of non-malignant conditions such as endometriosis, pregnancy or any inflammatory condition of the abdomen
> - Ovarian torsion may induce a massively elevated level

sample is obtained, further imaging with MRI would usually be unnecessary unless the biopsy shows features of malignancy.

The complex cystic mass could represent ovarian cancer and therefore should be evaluated further. A serum CA-125 level should be obtained in the first instance (Box 21.4). Further characterization of the lesion with an MRI examination of the pelvis would be very useful in this context.

Mrs Howell sees the gynaecologist who sends blood for a CA-125 level and performs a pipelle biopsy. At her follow-up appointment the following week, Mrs Howell is told that the CA-125 level is 15 IU/mL (within normal range).

Does the normal CA-125 level rule out ovarian cancer as the cause of the complex cystic mass?

No, an elevated CA-125 is only seen in 80% of cases of ovarian cancer. A normal level does not rule it out and hence it is of little value for screening asymptomatic

patients. Its value lies in monitoring patients' response to therapy by serial measurements in those cases where it is elevated.

However, the pipelle biopsy shows well-differentiated endometrial adenocarcinoma. In the light of these findings, an MRI examination of the pelvis is performed to: (1) stage the endometrial carcinoma, and (2) characterize the cystic ovarian lesion.

What does Fig. 21.5 show?

Figure 21.5 is a T1-weighted axial view of the pelvis. The complex cystic mass is demonstrated. The larger cystic component that was seen on ultrasound is seen in the centre of the image. Posterior to this, on the left, there is a hyperintense (bright) structure (Fig. 21.5, arrow).

What substances appear bright on T1-weighted imaging?

- Fat
- Gadolinium (i.e. contrast medium)
- Methaemoglobin (i.e. subacute haemorrhage)
- Proteinaceous fluid (including pus)
- Melanin
- Calcium (rare)

What does Fig. 21.6 show?

This is a T1-weighted fat-saturation image at the same level. In this type of sequence, the signal from fat is suppressed – instead of appearing hyperintense, fat appears hypointense. The structure indicated in Fig. 21.5 has become hypointense and is therefore predominantly composed of fat. The same structure is hyperintense in Fig. 21.7, a T2-weighted image of the same level. This would also be consistent with the presence of fat. Of note,

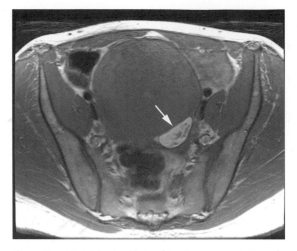

Figure 21.5 T1-weighted axial view from the MRI examination of the pelvis.

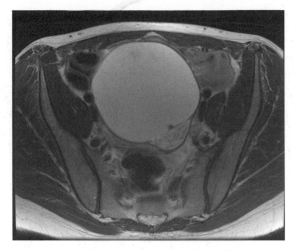

Figure 21.7 T2-weighted image from the MRI examination of the pelvis.

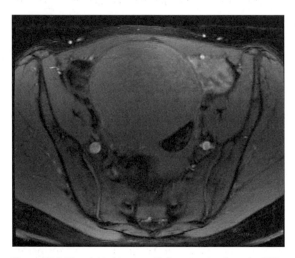

Figure 21.6 T1-weighted image with fat saturation from the MRI examination of the pelvis.

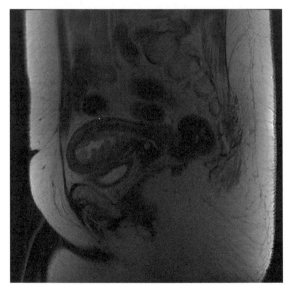

Figure 21.8 T2-weighted sagittal image from the MRI examination of the pelvis.

methaemoglobin may show an increase in signal on fat-saturated images.

How does this help?

The differential diagnosis for a complex cystic mass in the pelvis is very wide, ranging from benign cysts to frank ovarian cancer. However, a complex cystic mass containing fat is almost always an ovarian teratoma (also known as a dermoid cyst). These are almost always benign tumours, derived from pluripotential stem cells that form tissues from all three primordial germ cell layers.

They often contain variable amounts of fat, fluid, hair, cartilage, bone and even fully formed teeth.

What do the other images show?

Figures 21.8 and 21.9 are sagittal sections through the uterus. These are T2-weighted and T1-weighted following administration of intravenous gadolinium, respectively. The endometrium is thickened and there is invasion of tumour in to the myometrium. This invasion

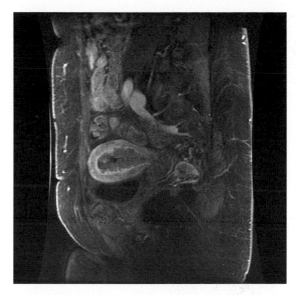

Figure 21.9 T1-weighted sagittal image from the MRI examination of the pelvis following administration of intravenous gadolinium.

> **Box 21.5 Staging of endometrial cancer**
>
> | | |
> |---|---|
> | IA | Tumour limited to endometrium |
> | IB | Tumour invades up to less than half of myometrium |
> | IC | Tumour invades to more than half of myometrium |
> | II | Tumour invades cervix but does not extend beyond uterus |
> | IIIA | Tumour invades the serosa or adnexa, or malignant peritoneal cytology |
> | IIIB | Vaginal involvement (direct extension or metastasis) |
> | IIIC | Metastasis to pelvic and/or para-aortic lymph nodes |
> | IVA | Tumour invades bladder mucosa and/or bowel mucosa |
> | IVB | Distant metastasis |

does not reach the serosal surface; neither the cervix nor adnexa are involved.

The radiologist diagnoses an ovarian teratoma based on the imaging characteristics described above. They also stage the endometrial cancer as IC (Box 21.5).

The radiological staging is important in that it determines the type of surgery. In early endometrial cancer, a transabdominal hysterectomy with bilateral salpingo-oophorectomy (removal of the uterus, fallopian tubes and ovaries) is performed. If the patient has only super-ficial invasion of the myometrium, the surgeon will often sample the pelvic lymph nodes. In more advanced disease, either deep invasion or enlarged pelvic lymph nodes on MRI, a formal lymph node dissection will be performed. Where possible, this is avoided as it is a more complex procedure with a higher risk of postoperative complications. In more advanced disease (stage III or IV), radiotherapy or chemotherapy is indicated.

After discussion at the multidisciplinary team meeting with the radiologist and histopathologist, the surgeon plans a transabdominal hysterectomy with bilateral salpingo-oophorectomy and lymph node dissection. She plans to remove the teratoma as part of the operation (obviously this would be removed with the ovary). Mrs Howell undergoes surgery and makes a good initial postoperative recovery. Surgical histology confirms stage IC disease and the pelvic lymph nodes are not involved.

Seven days after the operation, the ward doctor is called to see her as she is feeling short of breath. The ward doctor assesses her as follows:

Airway	*Patent; patient able to talk in short sentences*
Breathing	*Respiratory rate 22 breaths/minute*
	O_2 saturation 92% breathing room air
	Breath sounds normal, trachea central
Circulation	*Pulse 110 beats/minute, regular*
	Blood pressure 110/80 mmHg
	Heart sounds normal

Mrs Howell denies chest or abdominal pain. She is afebrile. She has never had any previous similar episodes.

What would you do next?

Mrs Howell is hypoxic. The first step should be to administer oxygen via a 60% Venturi mask to improve the oxygen saturation. An arterial blood gas sample should be taken. The advantage of a Venturi mask is that it delivers a controlled concentration of oxygen – arterial blood gas sampling can therefore be carried out while the patient is breathing oxygen.

What is the differential diagnosis of postoperative hypoxia?

Breathlessness following surgery is usually caused by one of the following:
- Infection
- Pulmonary embolism
- Pneumothorax, often complicating central venous line insertion

Box 21.6 Arterial blood gas results	
PO$_2$	11 kPa (on 60% O$_2$)
PCO$_2$	3.9 kPa
pH	7.44
Base excess	1 mmol/L

- Mucous plugging of the large airways, usually responds well to physiotherapy
- Fluid overload, may indicate an underlying myocardial infarction

The arterial blood gas results are given in Box 21.6.

What do the arterial blood gas results indicate?

The PO$_2$ is within the normal range for someone breathing air. Considering Mrs Howell is breathing 60% oxygen the PO$_2$ is very low. The PCO$_2$ is also low indicating a type 1 respiratory failure. The pH and base excess are within normal limits.

What would you do next?

Although many arterial blood gas analysers will provide results for a variety of blood tests including full blood count and urea and electrolytes, formal venous sample analysis is more accurate and should also be carried out.

Blood tests

- Full blood count – to look for anaemia (a postoperative bleed could be the cause of her breathlessness) or an inflammatory response (sepsis can make you breathless)
- Urea and electrolytes – to look for electrolyte imbalance
- C-reactive protein – to look for an inflammatory response
- D-dimers – these are breakdown products of fibrin often elevated in patients with thromboembolism. However, these are of no value in this situation as the recent surgery would also cause the result to be abnormal

ECG

Carried out to look for cardiac causes of breathlessness, e.g. a silent myocardial infarction. Specific ECG changes from pulmonary embolism are helpful if present, but are not often seen.

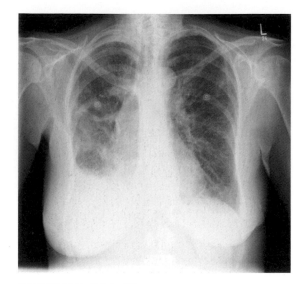

Figure 21.10 Frontal chest X-ray.

Chest X-ray

Chest X-ray to assess the lungs. In view of the patient's condition, it may be safest to request this be performed on the ward rather than sending the patient to the radiology department.

The blood tests were unremarkable. The ECG showed a sinus tachycardia only.

What does the image show?

Figure 21.10 shows Mrs Howell's chest X-ray. There is an area of consolidation in the right lower zone with obscuration of the right hemidiaphragm, indicating pathology involving the right lower lobe. This would be consistent with infection in the right clinical context. However, we know in this case that the inflammatory markers are normal and that she does not have a raised temperature. It should be remembered that consolidation simply represents opacification of the air spaces. Although commonly caused by infection, haemorrhage, oedema, and malignancy, a number of other conditions can cause consolidation.

What do you suspect could be the cause of the type I respiratory failure?

A patient who is 7 days post pelvic surgery who suddenly develops type I respiratory failure should have the diagnosis of pulmonary embolism actively excluded.

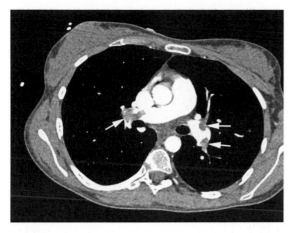

Figure 21.11 Axial CT image (soft tissue windows) through the thorax following administration of intravenous contrast medium.

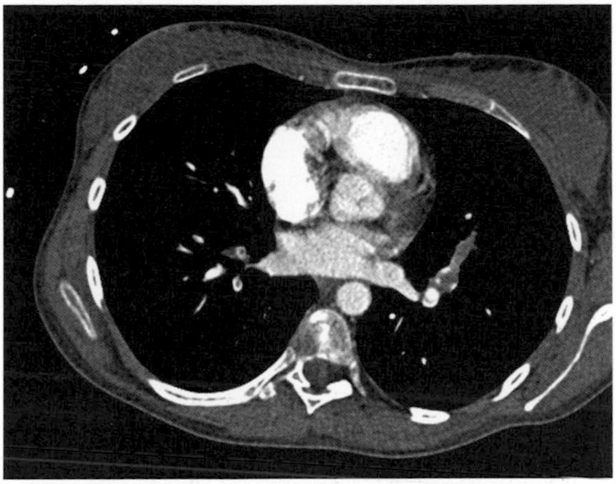

Figure 21.12 Axial CT image (soft tissue windows) through the thorax following administration of intravenous contrast medium.

How would you investigate further?

There are two principal imaging modalities for the investigation of suspected pulmonary embolism: CT (CT pulmonary angiogram [CTPA]) and nuclear medicine (ventilation–perfusion [V/Q] scintigraphy). In most departments, the decision as to which of the two should be used is most often decided by the chest X-ray and the clinical history. A V/Q scan is of value in patients with a normal chest X-ray in whom there is no pre-existing cardiorespiratory disease. It has a significant lower radiation burden to the patient (one-sixth that of a CTPA), but is not available out of hours. Alternatively, a CTPA may be performed; this directly visualizes the opacification of the pulmonary arteries. It allows the radiologist to also look for other causes of respiratory failure and may be performed at any time.

What do the images show?

The imaging is timed to coincide with the contrast medium opacifying the pulmonary arteries. These should appear as white branching vessels when viewed on soft tissue windows. The CTPA images in Figs 21.11 and 21.12 demonstrate filling defects (black areas; arrows) within both pulmonary arteries. These areas represent blood clots within the pulmonary arteries (i.e. multiple pulmonary emboli).

Mrs Howell was given treatment dose low molecular weight heparin initially and warfarin therapy was commenced. Once the warfarin was at a therapeutic level and her respiratory symptoms had subsided, she was discharged and made a good postoperative recovery. Mrs Howell continued on the warfarin for 6 months as this was her first pulmonary embolus.

CASE REVIEW

Jane Howell, a 69-year-old woman, presents to her GP with a 2-week history of postmenopausal bleeding. Abdominal and vaginal examinations are unremarkable. The GP takes blood samples and refers the patient to a one-stop clinic for post-menopausal bleeding.

She undergoes transabdominal and transvaginal ultrasound examinations of the abdomen and pelvis as part of her attendance at the one-stop clinic. A complex cystic mass is identified, as well as endometrial thickening. Mrs Howell is then seen by a gynaecologist who performs a pipelle biopsy.

The biopsy result is positive for endometrial cancer. The patient is referred for an MRI study, which demonstrates fat within the complex cystic pelvic mass, indicating that

Continued

this is a dermoid cyst. The endometrial cancer is staged during the same examination and is found to have deep myometrial invasion (stage IC).

In view of the findings, Mrs Howell undergoes transabdominal hysterectomy and bilateral salpingo-oophorectomy with pelvic lymph node dissection and makes a good initial postoperative recovery.

At 7 days after the operation, Mrs Howell becomes acutely short of breath. Arterial blood gas reveals a type 1 respiratory failure. Mrs Howell is investigated with blood tests, an ECG and a chest X-ray. Pulmonary embolism is suspected and a CTPA is requested which demonstrates multiple pulmonary emboli. The patient is anticoagulated and makes an uneventful recovery thereafter.

KEY POINTS

- Post-menopausal bleeding requires thorough investigation, either by a gynaecologist or at a 'one-stop' clinic
- Initial assessment should be with ultrasound
- If endometrial thickening is identified, tissue sampling should be undertaken
- Pelvic masses should be investigated with CA-125 and cross-sectional imaging, preferably MRI
- MRI characteristics can be diagnostic in the case of dermoid cysts
- Endometrial cancer should be staged with MRI to enable preoperative surgical planning
- Higher stage endometrial cancer requires pelvic lymph node dissection

- In patients with sudden onset shortness of breath, an arterial blood gas should be taken and oxygen administered
- Radiological investigation of suspected pulmonary embolism should start with a chest X-ray
- If the chest X-ray is normal, with no history of cardiorespiratory disease, then a V/Q scintigram should be requested
- If the chest X-ray is abnormal, there is pre-existing cardiorespiratory disease, the patient is very unwell or needs to be imaged out of hours, then a CTPA should be requested

Radiology: Clinical Cases Uncovered. By A. S. Shaw, E. M. Godfrey, A. Singh and T. F. Massoud. Published 2009 by Blackwell Publishing. ISBN 978-1-4051-8474-8.

Case 22 — A 30-year-old woman with right iliac fossa pain

Stephanie Neame, a 30-year-old woman, presents to the accident and emergency department one evening with severe right iliac fossa pain that had come on gradually during the day. On questioning, she said that the pain had not moved around the abdomen. It made her feel nauseated but she had not been vomiting. Indeed, Stephanie had not been able to eat anything because of this pain and nausea all day. She had opened her bowels normally that morning and had no urinary symptoms. She had no significant past medical, surgical or family history. She lives with her boyfriend who is well.

What questions would you ask for a basic gynaecological history?

The key features in a gynaecological history are detailed in Box 22.1.

Stephanie denies any vaginal discharge but admits to occasional dyspareunia. She does not think she is likely to be pregnant because she takes the oral contraceptive pill, and has never been pregnant.

On examination she is found to be afebrile, has a pulse of 90 beats/minute and a blood pressure of 120/80 mmHg. Her heart and breath sounds are normal. There is moderate tenderness in her right iliac fossa with rebound tenderness. Digital rectal examination is unremarkable, but vaginal examination revealed some tenderness in the right adnexa and cervical excitation; no masses were palpable.

What is cervical excitation?

Cervical excitation is pain associated with gentle movement of the cervix during bi-manual vaginal examination. There are a number of causes including ectopic pregnancy, pelvic infections and endometriosis.

What is the differential diagnosis of acute right iliac fossa pain?

The differential for acute right iliac fossa pain in young men is rather narrow:
- Appendicitis
- Diverticulitis
- Epiploic appendagitis (Box 22.2 and Fig. 22.1)
- Mesenteric adenitis
- Crohn's disease

In young women the differential is wider and includes gynaecological causes:
- Ectopic pregnancy
- Endometriosis
- Pelvic inflammatory disease such as:
  - oophoritis
  - salpingitis
  - cervicitis
  - endometritis

In older patients of either sex, colorectal cancer should also be considered.

What investigations would you arrange at this point?

- Urinary beta human chorionic gonadotrophin (β-HCG) – although Stephanie thinks she is unlikely to be pregnant as she is taking the oral contraceptive pill, a pregnancy test (with her consent) is essential. No method of contraception is infallible
- Urine dipstick – to exclude a urinary tract infection
- Full blood count (FBC) – the neutrophil count may be raised in infection
- C-reactive protein (CRP) – may be raised in infection or inflammation

The urinary pregnancy test and dipstick were both negative. The neutrophil count was raised at 9.5 and the CRP was also raised at 78. The neutrophils showed 'left shift', suggestive of inflammation.

155

Box 22.1 Important questions in a gynaecological history

Regarding the acute episode:
- Is there any vaginal discharge?
- Do you experience any pain during sexual intercourse (dyspareunia)?
  Regarding the medical history:
- Is there any chance you could be pregnant?
- Do you use contraception, and if so what type?
- How many pregnancies have you had?
- How many children have you had?

Box 22.2 Epiploic appendagitis

Epiploic appendagitis is an unusual self-limiting inflammation of one of the epiploic appendages. These are sausage-shaped fat-filled pouches of peritoneum that arise in intervals from the surface of the entire colon.

Appendagitis may arise because of torsion or venous thrombosis. When it occurs on the right side it may clinically mimic acute appendicitis; on the left side, diverticulitis. The diagnosis is usually made on CT; an example is shown in Fig. 22.1. The radiological hallmark at CT is of a fat density structure, adjacent to the colon, surrounded by soft tissue density stranding.

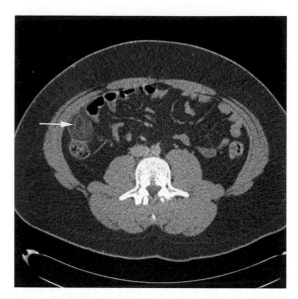

Figure 22.1 Axial CT image demonstrating epiploic appendagitis (arrow).

If the FBC and CRP were normal, would appendicitis remain a possibility?

Yes, unfortunately a normal full blood count and CRP does not exclude appendicitis. A commonly used clinical scoring system is the Alvarado scoring system (Box 22.3).

According to the Alvarado system, Stephanie scored 8 (2 points for right iliac fossa tenderness and a raised neutrophil count and 1 point each for nausea, anorexia, rebound tenderness and left shift). This score makes appendicitis probable.

Box 22.3 Alvarado scoring system for acute appendicitis

Migratory right iliac fossa pain	1 point
Anorexia	1 point
Nausea or vomiting	1 point
Right iliac fossa tenderness	2 points
Rebound tenderness	1 point
Pyrexia	1 point
Raised white cell count	2 points
Neutrophils showing left shift (a blood film indicator of a bone marrow response to acute illness, often inflammation)	1 point

Score	Interpretation
1–4	Appendicitis is unlikely
5–6	Equivocal
7–8	Appendicitis probable
9–10	Appendicitis highly likely

Would you arrange any imaging at this point, and if so, what?

Many patients presenting with right iliac fossa pain will not require imaging. This particularly applies to male patients because the only life-threatening frequently occurring condition is appendicitis. The diagnosis of 'appendicitis or not' in men can often be made clinically.

In women the decision is more difficult. As outlined above, the crucial first step is to perform a pregnancy test to identify those women who could potentially have an ectopic pregnancy. Women with a positive test should undergo immediate ultrasound and be closely monitored by a gynaecologist.

In women with a negative pregnancy test, the decision whether to request an ultrasound examination is based on the overall clinical condition of the patient. The more

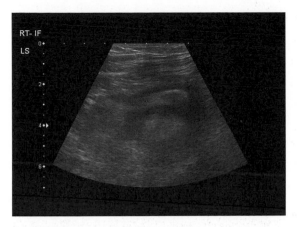

Figure 22.2 Ultrasound image of the pelvis.

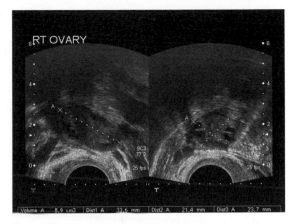

Figure 22.4 Ultrasound image of the pelvis.

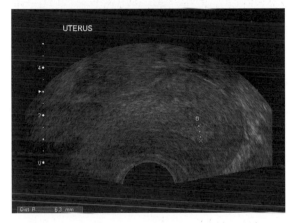

Figure 22.3 Ultrasound image of the pelvis.

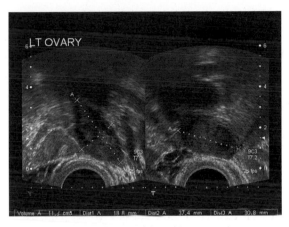

Figure 22.5 Ultrasound image of the pelvis.

unwell and septic a patient is, the more likely an ultrasound will be useful, and the sooner it should be performed.

In those patients, male or female, with an atypical presentation, a CT examination may be required as this gives a more general survey of the abdomen and pelvis. However, ionizing radiation should be avoided whenever possible.

An ultrasound examination was requested to assess the gynaecological organs and to look for an inflamed appendix.

What do the images show?

Figure 22.2 is an ultrasound image showing a blind-ending thick-walled tubular structure in the right iliac fossa. This would be strongly suggestive of appendicitis. Figures 22.3–22.5 show a healthy uterus and ovaries.

What would be better for the patient – an open or laparoscopic appendicectomy?

There are a number of advantages and disadvantages for each technique. These are summarized in Box 22.4. In general, for young women, the laparoscopic approach is preferred. This is partly for cosmetic reasons, but also because it allows the ovaries to be inspected more closely (this is obviously more important if the patient does not undergo preoperative ultrasound).

Stephanie undergoes a laparoscopic appendicectomy the same evening. On inspection, the appendix was inflamed, and this was later confirmed on histological analysis. She is discharged the following day and makes a good recovery.

Box 22.4 Comparison of laparoscopic with open appendicectomy

	Open	**Laparoscopic**
Cost	Cheaper	More expensive
Cosmesis	Worse	Better
Ability to review rest of abdominal contents	Worse	Better
Wound infection rate	Worse	Better
Postoperative abdominal collection rate	Better	Worse
Return to work	Same	Same

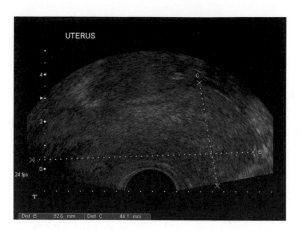

Figure 22.6 Transvaginal ultrasound image of the uterus.

Two years later, Stephanie re-presents to the accident and emergency department with right iliac fossa pain. On close questioning, Stephanie feels that this episode, although severe, is different to the pain she had during her previous attendance. She describes previous cyclical episodes of less severe pain over the previous year. In addition, she has had dyspareunia and irregular menstrual bleeding. She denies urinary or bowel symptoms. She continues to take the oral contraceptive pill.

On examination there is deep tenderness in the right iliac fossa, but no rebound or percussion tenderness. Digital rectal examination is normal. On vaginal examination there is again cervical excitation and right adnexal tenderness. Temperature, pulse and blood pressure are normal. The admitting doctor arranges a β-HCG, FBC and CRP which are normal.

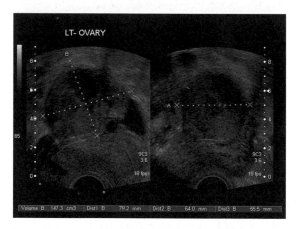

Figure 22.7 Transvaginal ultrasound image of the left ovary.

What imaging would you arrange?

This presentation is fairly similar to the previous episode, although the cyclical nature of the pain makes a gynae-cological cause rather more likely (as does the previous appendicectomy). An ultrasound of the pelvis would therefore be a useful test, as before.

What do the images show?

Figure 22.6 demonstrates a normal uterus in longitudinal section. Figures 22.7 and 22.8 demonstrate both ovaries (each image comprises two perpendicular views) and their dimensions. Both ovaries are seen to be massively enlarged; the normal ovarian volume in a woman of reproductive age is less than 15 mL. In this case, the left ovary has a volume of 147 mL (diameter 79 mm) and the right ovary 159 mL (diameter 88 mm).

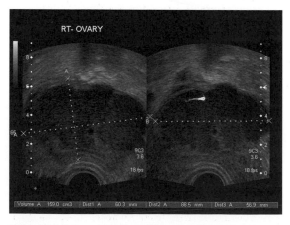

Figure 22.8 Transvaginal ultrasound image of the right ovary.

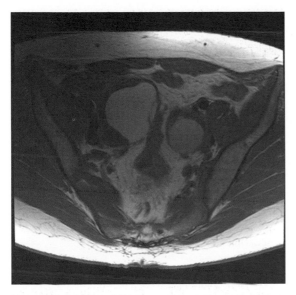

Figure 22.9 Axial T1-weighted image through the ovarian lesions.

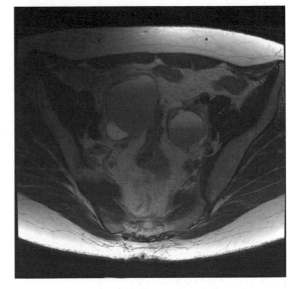

Figure 22.10 Axial T2-weighted image through the ovarian lesions.

> **Box 22.5 Substances that appear bright on T1-weighted MRI**
>
> - Fat
> - Gadolinium (contrast medium)
> - Subacute haemorrhage (methaemoglobin)
> - Protein-rich fluid
> - Melanin
> - Particulate calcium

What might be the cause of these ovarian lesions?

Possible causes of bilateral enlarged ovaries include:

- Solid:
  - endometriomas (endometriosis deposits)
  - Krukenberg tumours (bilateral metastases that reach the ovaries via transcoelomic spread – often from a gastric tumour)
  - bilateral oophoritis (as part of pelvic inflammatory disease)
  - ovarian carcinoma
- Cystic:
  - polycystic ovary syndrome
  - ovarian hyperstimulation syndrome (usually during fertility treatment)

The ovaries do not appear cystic here, so the cause is likely one of the first three given. Of these, oophoritis would be unlikely here given the normal FBC and CRP on admission.

What imaging would be appropriate next?

Endometriosis is best imaged with pelvic MRI, whereas a CT of the chest, abdomen and pelvis would be more appropriate if malignancy is suspected. An upper gastro-intestinal endoscopy would be required to look for gastric cancer. The choice between MRI and CT rests on which would be the most likely: endometriosis or Krukenberg tumours. Given Stephanie's age (32 at this point), the former is much more likely.

Stephanie is discharged with appropriate analgesia and an appointment for an outpatient MRI of the pelvis.

What do the images show?

The images show masses within each ovary. In Fig. 22.9, one can see that these masses are homogeneous and have high signal intensity (bright) on T1-weighted imaging. Box 22.5 lists the relatively few substances that are high signal on T1-weighted MRI.

Figure 22.10 is a standard T2-weighted image. On T2-weighted images fat appears as high signal, as does fluid. In order to differentiate the two, a variety of techniques may be used to suppress the signal from the fat. If both standard and fat-saturated T2-weighted sequences are obtained, it is possible to differentiate between fat and water. This is particularly useful in the diagnosis of adnexal lesions – fat-containing masses are very

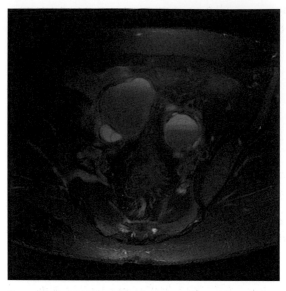

Figure 22.11 Axial T2-weighted fat-saturated image through the ovarian lesions.

likely to be dermoid cysts, as seen in the previous case. Furthermore, fat-saturated images make fluid more conspicuous.

The masses shown here are bright on both standard and fat-saturated T2-weighted sequences (Fig. 22.11), implying that they contain fluid.

The images show masses that are bright on T1-weighted imaging, but are not fat. What is the diagnosis?

There is one final clue – the layering of signal intensity seen on both T2-weighted sequences is known as 'shading'. It occurs when extracellular methaemoglobin (high signal) layers on top of haemosiderin (low signal). This sign is pathognomonic of endometriomas. Endometriomas (also known as 'chocolate' cysts because of the dark brown colour of the altered blood which they contain) are focal deposits of endometriosis.

Endometriosis can be defined as the presence of endometrial tissue outside the uterus. There are a number of theories as to how endometriosis develops, some of which are discussed in Box 22.6. Endometriosis most commonly affects the pelvis, but other sites of disease may be seen (Box 22.7).

Stephanie has the diagnosis of endometriosis explained to her by the gynaecologist. He outlines the treatment options (Box 22.8). Stephanie decides to try medical therapy in the first instance and is given a follow-up appointment.

Box 22.6 Theories about endometriosis

Metastatic theory
- Fragments of endometrial tissue detach and spread directly to various sites around the peritoneum via retrograde menstruation
- In order to explain the presence of endometrial tissue in sites distant to the peritoneum, such as the brain, haematological spread would also be required

Metaplastic theory
- Coelomic metaplasia, in which stem cells are stimulated by an unknown factor to develop in to endometrial tissue

Induction theory
- An unidentified factor (hereditary or environmental) is responsible for causing transformation of normal tissue in to ectopic endometrial tissue

Hormone imbalance
- Excess oestrogen
- Low progesterone levels

Box 22.7 Disease sites for endometriosis and symptoms

- *Reproductive tract:* pelvic pain, abnormal menstruation, urinary symptoms, infertility
- *Gastrointestinal tract:* catamenial diarrhoea, constipation, rectal pain or bleeding
- *Urinary tract:* catamenial urgency, frequency, and haematuria; urinary obstruction or flank pain
- *Chest:* catamenial haemoptysis, pleuritic chest pain or pneumothorax
- *Cutaneous tissue:* catamenial bleeding, palpable mass
- *Central nervous system:* catamenial headaches or seizures

Box 22.8 Therapeutic options in endometriosis

- Medical:
  ○ pain relief (NSAIDs also reduce menstrual flow)
  ○ hormone manipulation
- Surgical:
  ○ resection or ablation of endometriotic tissue
  ○ hysterectomy and bilateral salpingo-oophorectomy is the definitive treatment
  ○ bowel resection, where symptoms dictate
  ○ pre-sacral neurectomy, may help severe pelvic pain

CASE REVIEW

A 30-year-old woman presents to the accident and emergency department with severe right iliac fossa pain, fever and raised inflammatory markers. She undergoes ultrasound which indicates that she has acute appendicitis. She undergoes laparoscopic appendicectomy and makes an uneventful recovery.

Approximately 2 years later, she re-presents to the accident and emergency department with a subjectively different, cyclical right iliac fossa pain which has become acutely worse. Her inflammatory markers are normal. She again undergoes ultrasound which demonstrates bilaterally enlarged ovaries with a normal uterus.

She subsequently undergoes MRI study of the pelvis. This confirms that the ovarian lesions comprise blood and a diagnosis of endometriosis is made.

KEY POINTS

- The gynaecological history is important in young women
- Female patients of childbearing age presenting with abdominal pain must have a pregnancy test
- Epiploic appendagitis is an unusual cause of right iliac fossa pain, usually diagnosed on CT
- Pelvic ultrasound is a useful investigation in women with right iliac fossa pain; the ovaries and appendix can often be readily visualized

- Appendicitis is not excluded by normal inflammatory markers
- Appendicectomy may be either laparoscopic or open; there are advantages and disadvantages with each approach
- Endometriosis is best diagnosed with pelvic MRI, but may manifest in many ways according to the site of disease

Case 23 A 75-year-old man with back pain

Mr Samuel Allsopp, a 75-year-old man, presents to his GP with sudden onset upper lumbar back pain radiating to his abdomen. The pain is severe and started that morning. He has not had back pain before and there is no history of trauma. He is a 30 pack-year ex-smoker with a past medical history of chronic obstructive pulmonary disease (COPD) for which he is occasionally admitted to hospital. He takes inhaled steroids and ipratropium for his COPD and has no allergies. He has no significant family history and lives at home with his wife who is well. They have a good quality of life together. He denies bladder or bowel symptoms.

What are you concerned about here?

Lumbar back pain is a very common complaint. In the vast majority of patients with lumbar back pain, the cause will be musculoskeletal degenerative change. This group responds well to simple measures such as keeping active, weight loss and analgesia. GPs face the difficult task of differentiating the few patients with more worrying pathology from this large group. One of the ways they do this is by asking the patient about so-called 'red flag symptoms' (Box 23.1).

Importantly, the 'red flag' symptoms described in Box 23.1 are only applicable to chronic back pain. Mr Allsopp had a sudden onset of back pain with no previous episodes, which in itself is concerning. Points that should be considered during the examination are:

• Lumbar disc herniation
• Pathological fracture (e.g. caused by osteoporosis secondary to steroid treatment of COPD)
• Leaking abdominal aortic aneurysm (AAA)
• Pancreatitis

• Spinal abscess
• Spinal tumour
• Spinal subarachnoid haemorrhage (rare)

The GP examines Mr Allsopp and finds him to be sweaty, pale and unwell. There is epigastric tenderness and a pulsatile mass. Peripheral nerve examination of the lower limbs is unremarkable.

What would you do now?

There is a good chance that Mr Allsopp could have a leaking AAA. This is a surgical emergency. It is imperative that he is transferred as quickly as possible to hospital for appropriate imaging and assessment by a vascular surgeon.

The GP makes a provisional diagnosis of leaking AAA. She therefore calls 999 for an ambulance and while waiting for it to arrive inserts two large-bore intravenous cannulae, taking blood samples at the same time to send with the patient to hospital.

What blood samples should the GP take?

• Full blood count – as a baseline, and to assess for possible blood loss
• Clotting screen – to look for a bleeding diathesis
• Urea and electrolytes – to assess renal function
• Cross-match – to provide blood for resuscitation

The ambulance arrives and takes Mr Allsopp to hospital. The GP telephones Mrs Allsopp to explain what has happened.

At the accident and emergency department the admitting doctor sends the blood samples obtained by the GP to the haematology and biochemistry department. He immediately reviews Mr Allsopp as he is concerned that he may be shocked.

Radiology: Clinical Cases Uncovered. By A. S. Shaw, E. M. Godfrey, A. Singh and T. F. Massoud. Published 2009 by Blackwell Publishing. ISBN 978-1-4051-8474-8.

What is the definition of shock and what are the different types?

Shock can be defined as insufficient circulation to perfuse the tissues adequately. There are a variety of different types, each with several causes – these are summarized in Box 23.2. The most likely cause in this case is hypovolaemic shock secondary to blood loss within the abdomen.

How do you assess whether a patient is shocked?

The assessment of whether a patient is shocked is clinical. There are no blood tests; imaging findings are late and unreliable. The crucial things to assess are:

- Pulse
- Blood pressure
- Capillary refill
- Respiratory rate
- Urine output

The American College of Surgeons have described four stages of shock, as detailed in Box 23.3. This table is an important one for two reasons. First, it is a guide to which features are reliable indicators of early shock (note

that systolic blood pressure is unlikely to alter until more than 30% of the blood volume has been lost). Secondly, the stage of shock determines what should be used for volume replacement. Crystalloids alone are suitable for stage I and II shock, but should be combined with blood for stages III and IV.

Fluid resuscitation in suspected leaking AAA is complicated by the need to maintain a relatively low blood pressure to reduce the risk of complete rupture. Although no good quality evidence exists to guide fluid resuscitation in this context, many experts suggest that one should aim to maintain the systolic pressure at about 100 mmHg.

Box 23.1 'Red flag' symptoms in chronic lumbar back pain

- Thoracic pain
- Fever and unexplained weight loss
- Bladder or bowel dysfunction
- History of carcinoma
- Ill health or presence of other medical illness
- Progressive neurological deficit
- Disturbed gait, saddle anaesthesia
- Age of onset <20 years or >55 years

Box 23.2 Types of shock

- Hypovolaemic:
  - blood loss
  - dehydration (e.g. in vomiting or diarrhoea)
- Cardiogenic:
  - myocardial infarction
  - arrhythmias
  - myocarditis
- Distributive:
  - anaphylactic: e.g. peanuts (true anaphylaxis); intravenous contrast medium (an anaphylactoid reaction)
  - septic
  - neurogenic (e.g. spinal trauma)
- Obstructive:
  - pulmonary embolism
  - tension pneumothorax
  - cardiac tamponade
- Endocrine:
  - acute adrenal insufficiency

Box 23.3 Severity of shock, taken from the ATLS Manual (American College of Surgeons)

	Class I	Class II	Class III	Class IV
Blood loss (mL)	<750	750–1500	1500–2000	>2000
Blood loss (% blood volume)	<15%	15–30%	30–40%	>40%
Pulse	<100	>100	>120	>140
Blood pressure	Normal	Normal	Decreased	Decreased
Pulse pressure	Normal or increased	Decreased	Decreased	Decreased
Respiratory rate	14–20	20–30	30–40	>35
Urine output (mL/hr)	>30	20–30	5–15	Negligible
CNS	Slightly anxious	Mildly anxious	Anxious, confused	Confused lethargic
Fluid replacement	Crystalloid	Crystalloid	Crystalloid and blood	Crystalloid and blood

The admitting doctor finds the following in his assessment of Mr Allsopp:

Airway	Patent; patient able to talk
Breathing	Chest clear
	Trachea central
	Respiratory rate 30 breaths/minute
Circulation	Capillary refill delayed
	Jugular venous pressure not visible
	Heart sounds normal
	Pulse 122 beats/minute
	Blood pressure 80/60 mm Hg
Disposition	Anxious

The admitting doctor diagnoses class III shock and commences fluid resuscitation with normal saline. He also administers high flow oxygen and telephones the blood bank in the haematology department to ask for type-specific blood. Box 23.4 describes the different ways of obtaining blood for transfusion in emergencies. A urinary catheter is inserted to monitor urine output.

After abdominal examination the admitting doctor feels that the GP's provisional diagnosis is likely correct and calls the vascular surgeon to the accident and emergency department. The vascular surgeon reassesses Mr Alssopp and finds the following:

Capillary refill delayed
Pulse 100 beats/minute
Blood pressure 100/80 mm Hg

Box 23.4 Methods for obtaining blood for transfusion in an emergency

- The quickest way of obtaining blood in an emergency is to ask for O negative blood. This can be given to patients without cross-matching and is therefore available immediately. A supply is often kept in the accident and emergency and surgical departments. There is a limited supply so its use is reserved for patients who cannot wait for type-specific or fully cross-matched blood
- Type-specific blood can be obtained from the transfusion department relatively quickly (in about 15 minutes). It has the advantage of being available more quickly than fully cross-matched blood and is in more plentiful supply than O negative blood (assuming the recipient is not O negative)
- Fully cross-matching blood takes approximately 1 hour. This may not be possible in an emergency. If at all possible cross-matched blood should be used as antibody-mediated transfusion reactions are much less likely

---

The vascular surgeon feels that Mr Allsopp is responding to fluid resuscitation and is therefore stable enough for imaging. The type-specific blood transfusion is started.

What image modality would be used here?

Ultrasound in the accident and emergency department could be used to confirm the presence of an AAA but would not be able to determine whether it is leaking. The best test here would be an abdominal CT examination. This would be able to detect the presence of an AAA as well as whether or not it was leaking. One can also determine the location of the aneurysm with respect to the vascular branches of the abdominal aorta.

What are the branches of the abdominal aorta?

Box 23.5 summarizes the various branches of the abdominal aorta.

Mr Allsopp undergoes a CT of the abdomen and pelvis.

What do the images show?

The axial CT images in Figs 23.1 and 23.2 show a dilated aorta with soft tissue stranding around it. This is an aortic aneurysm with blood leaking in to the retroperitoneal space causing soft tissue stranding.

Figure 23.1 is an unenhanced image, acquired before intravenous injection of contrast medium. The second image (Fig. 23.2) is in the arterial phase (approximately

---

Box 23.5 Branches of the abdominal aorta

Unpaired anterior branches
- Coeliac axis (arises at T12)
- Superior mesenteric artery (L1)
- Inferior mesenteric artery (L3)
- Median sacral artery (L4)

Paired lateral branches
- Subcostal arteries
- Inferior phrenic arteries
- Adrenal arteries
- Renal arteries (L2)
- Gonadal arteries
- Lumbar arteries (usually four pairs)
- Common iliac arteries (L4)

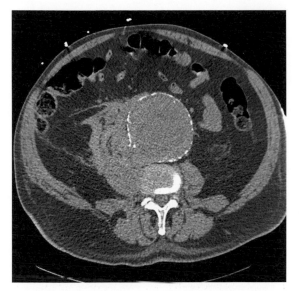

Figure 23.1 Axial CT image of the abdomen.

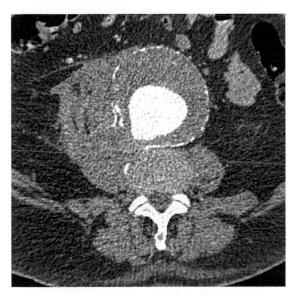

Figure 23.2 Axial CT image of the abdomen.

25–30 seconds following the intravenous injection), because most of the administered contrast medium is within the aorta rather than the inferior vena cava.

What is the definition of an aneurysm?

An aneurysm is a localized dilatation of an artery.

• True aneurysms involve all three layers of the vessel wall (tunica intima, tunica media and tunica adventitia). True aneurysms may be:

PART 2: CASES

> ### Box 23.6 Abdominal aortic aneurysms
>
> **Definition**
> Dilatation of the abdominal aorta to greater than 3 cm in antero-posterior diameter. Most common in elderly white males. Major risk factors include smoking, hypertension and a positive family history
>
> **Management**
> Asymptomatic aneurysms that are larger than 5 cm are considered for elective treatment. Smaller asymptomatic aneurysms are followed up with ultrasound or CT. Asymptomatic aneurysms are treated more aggressively as they are more likely to rupture (with the exception of inflammatory aneurysms). As the aneurysm enlarges, then the likelihood of it rupturing increases dramatically. According to Laplace's law, wall tension is proportional to the radius of the vessel
>
> **Causes**
> 1 Degenerative/atherosclerotic – the most common type by far
> 2 Inflammatory – more likely to be symptomatic but less likely to rupture. Erythrocyte sedimentation rate is raised. Surgery is more difficult
> 3 Mycotic (infected) – usually bacterial rather than fungal as the name implies, uncommon
> 4 Connective tissue disorders – e.g. Ehlers–Danlos or Marfan
> 5 Syphilis – rare
> Ninety-five per cent of AAAs are infrarenal and therefore treatable with surgery or endovascular repair. To anchor either type of graft, a cuff of infrarenal aortic wall is required. This is because the renal arteries cannot be sacrificed, unlike for example the inferior mesenteric artery

  ○ fusiform (spindle-shaped)
  ○ saccular
• False aneurysms are not contained by the vessel wall and are usually the result of trauma. They may be:
  ○ simple
  ○ complex (made up of multiple interconnecting cavities)
  Box 23.6 describes abdominal aortic aneurysms.

What type of image is this?

Figure 23.3 is a three-dimensional image that has been reconstructed in the coronal plane from the CT data to show the relationship of the aneurysm to the branches of the abdominal aorta. These are reviewed routinely prior

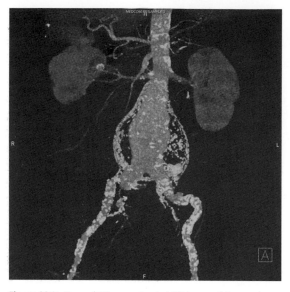

Figure 23.3   Coronal 3D reconstructed CT image of the abdominal aortic aneurysm.

to treatment. They provide a useful way of visualizing the anatomy of the aneurysm.

Is the aneurysm infrarenal (commencing below the level of the renal arteries)?

Yes – this means that operative management can be considered, either with open surgery or with an endovascular aneurysm repair (EVAR). The renal arteries are an important landmark as the surgeon will need to clamp the aorta below the renal artery and the interventional radiologist needs to place the superior end of the stent in normal calibre aorta below the renal arteries. Occluding a renal artery will lead to infarction of that kidney.

How should the patient be managed?

There are two major decisions to be made:

1 Should the patient be treated operatively or medically?
2 Should the patient be treated with surgery or EVAR?

In general, most patients with a leaking AAA will be offered operative treatment unless they are deemed unable to tolerate the procedure or if they have other significant coexisting medical conditions. Given Mr Allsopp's good quality of life and relatively young age, he would be managed operatively.

The question of surgery vs. EVAR is a difficult one. In the context of a leaking aneurysm, some patients may

> **Box 23.7 Endovascular aortic repair**
>
> EVAR is used in the elective and emergency treatment of AAA. Both femoral arteries are accessed via a surgical 'cut-down'. A wire is placed across the aneurysm and the collapsed stent is fed over the wire. The position is checked under fluoroscopy and the stent is then deployed, expanding to fit across the inside of the aneurysm and seal it at both ends.
>
> Sometimes, the stent will need to extend down in to an iliac artery and be combined with a femoral cross-over graft. In such cases, the contralateral iliac artery may need to be occluded to prevent filling of the aneurysm sac from below.
>
> The main advantage of EVAR over open surgical treatment is reduced postoperative morbidity. The main disadvantage is the annual follow-up with CT for the rest of the patient's life.

need to proceed directly to theatre for surgical control of the aorta. Those stable enough for imaging may be considered for EVAR, which has the advantage of reduced immediate postoperative morbidity.

Mr Allsopp's condition remains stable. The vascular surgeon discusses the case with an interventional radiologist. After reviewing the CT examination together the interventional radiologist agrees to perform an EVAR. Box 23.7 describes the key features of EVAR.

Mr Allsopp made a good postoperative recovery and returned home after 4 days. He returns for annual follow-up with CT.

What do the images show?

Figure 23.4 shows the CT topogram (scout view) with the EVAR graft *in situ*. Figure 23.5 is an unenhanced axial CT image demonstrating the aneurysm sac, within which is the graft (seen as a high attenuation dotted circle). Figure 23.6 is an arterial phase image at the same level demonstrating flow within the graft. There is additional contrast medium outside the graft (Fig. 23.6, arrow).

What is the significance of Fig. 23.6?

The presence of contrast medium outside the lumen of the graft indicates that there is an endoleak present. An endoleak is defined as a leak of blood (or contrast medium) outside the graft but within the aneurysm sac.

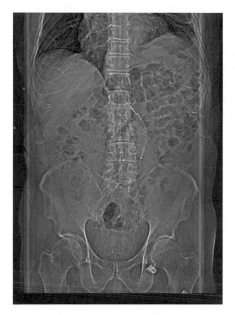

Figure 23.4 CT image of the abdomen following EVAR.

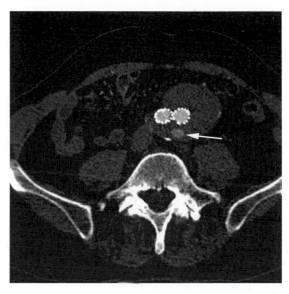

Figure 23.6 CT image of the abdomen following EVAR.

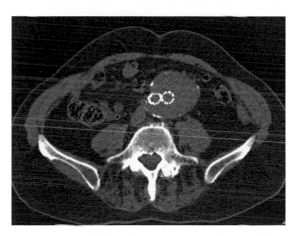

Figure 23.5 CT image of the abdomen following EVAR.

They are classified in to various different types because management depends on the cause of the leak (Box 23.8).

The radiologist reporting the CT notes the presence of the endoleak. He plans to perform conventional angiography to determine the type of endoleak, as the cause is not apparent on the CT examination.

This digital subtraction angiogram (DSA) image shows the endograft *in situ* (Fig. 23.7). There is contrast medium flow through it. The endoleak is again demonstrated but no connection with either end of the graft is apparent.

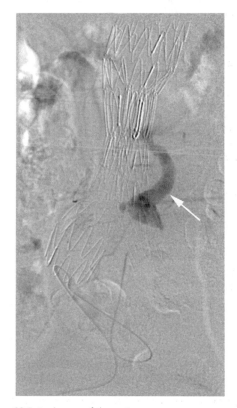

Figure 23.7 Angiogram of the aorta.

Box 23.8 Endoleak classification

Endoleak is usually detected on follow-up CT examinations. The cause may be apparent on the CT examination, but more commonly a conventional angiogram is required.

- Type I – Ineffective seal:
  - A – proximal
  - B – distal
  - C – iliac occluder
- Type II – Collateral flow:
  - A – single vessel
  - B – two or more vessels
- Type III – Structural failure:
  - A – junctional separation
  - B – endograft fracture or holes
- Type IV – Porosity of graft material
- Type V – Endotension (enlarging aneurysm sac under pressure but no obvious leak)

Box 23.9 Endoleak management

- Type I – Endovascular repair if possible.
- Type II:
  - shrinking aneurysmal sack – observe only
  - stable aneurysmal sack – controversial, but probably observe only
  - enlarging aneurysmal sack – endovascular repair
- Type III – Endovascular repair if possible
- Type IV – Observe only
- Type V – Optimal management remains unclear

There is no defect in the graft either. This endoleak is therefore a type II endoleak (often a diagnosis of exclusion).

The type II endoleak was managed conservatively by the clinical team (Box 23.9). The patient returned to annual follow-up and the endoleak resolved spontaneously over the next year.

CASE REVIEW

Samuel Allsopp, a 75-year-old man, presents to his GP with sudden onset back pain. The GP examines him and finds him to be unwell with a pulsatile expansile epigastric mass. The GP, suspecting a leaking AAA, calls an ambulance to take him to the accident and emergency department. While waiting, the GP inserts large-bore intravenous cannulae and takes blood samples.

The patient is assessed by the admitting physician who identifies shock and starts fluid resuscitation. Type-specific blood is obtained for concurrent transfusion and a urinary catheter is inserted. Clinically, the patient responds with a falling pulse and rising blood pressure. After assessment by a vascular surgeon, a CT examination of the abdomen and pelvis is requested.

The CT examination demonstrates a leaking AAA. The vascular surgeon refers the patient to an interventional radiologist who performs an EVAR. The patient makes an uncomplicated recovery.

A follow-up CT at 1 year demonstrates the presence of an endoleak. This is further assessed with conventional angiography, which confirms a type II endoleak. The patient is managed conservatively and the endoleak resolves spontaneously.

KEY POINTS

- Sudden onset severe back pain is a concerning symptom that requires prompt evaluation
- A suspected leaking AAA requires emergency transfer to hospital for assessment
- Hypovolaemic shock should be rapidly treated with intravenous crystalloid infusion +/– blood
- The imaging modality of choice for suspected leaking aneurysm is CT
- Leaking AAA may be treated with either open surgery or EVAR

- Open surgery is used in patients too unstable for EVAR, or for those with unsuitable anatomy
- Patients undergoing EVAR are followed up with annual CT for the rest of their lives
- Endoleak is defined as the leakage of blood outside the endograft but inside the aneurysmal sac
- The management of an endoleak depends on its type

A 30-year-old man with headache

Simon Black, a 30-year-old nurse, presents in the early evening to his local accident and emergency department with a severe headache. He walked in holding his head, accompanied by his wife who had driven him to hospital. On questioning, it seems that Simon had been out running after work and was having a shower when the headache started. Asked to describe it in more detail, he said that over the course of a minute or so he had developed the most severe headache he has ever experienced and that it was over his entire head. He described it as 'one of the worst things' he has ever experienced and thought he was going to die. Since the headache had started he had felt dizzy and nauseated. His wife adds that Simon was very unsteady on his feet and needed support to get in to the car. On arriving at the hospital, Mr Black had vomited in the car park. He has yet to take any analgesia for the headache.

What is the name given to this type of severe headache?

This is termed a 'thunderclap' headache because of its sudden onset.

What is the significance of this?

Some thunderclap headaches come on for no apparent reason. However, a number of medical emergencies may present with this sign including:
• Subarachnoid haemorrhage
• Cerebral aneurysm
• Intracranial arterial dissection
• Obstruction to the flow of cerebrospinal fluid (CSF)
• Pituitary infarction or haemorrhage
• Meningitis or encephalitis

Radiology: Clinical Cases Uncovered. By A. S. Shaw, E. M. Godfrey, A. Singh and T. F. Massoud. Published 2009 by Blackwell Publishing. ISBN 978-1-4051-8474-8.

What other points in the history may be relevant?
• Previous episodes
• Other medical conditions
• Family history
• Trauma

Mr Black mentions that he saw his family doctor a few weeks ago following two similar but less severe episodes of headache which had settled without treatment. He was told it could be a migraine or tension headache, particularly as his blood pressure was raised. The GP had prescribed some analgesics but not any anti-migraine medication. Simon is otherwise a fit and active amateur sportsman with no past medical history, although he had smoked for 5 years from the age of 16. Currently, the headache persists but is not as severe as when it first began.

On examination Mr Black is apyrexial but appears sweaty, pale and distressed. During the examination he asks the doctor to switch off some lights in the cubicle as he was finding them very uncomfortable. He is found to be tachycardic with a pulse rate of 110 beats/minute, and hypertensive with a blood pressure of 170/93 mmHg. The remainder of the cardiorespiratory system was normal. A thorough neurological examination was performed. Simon had features of meningism but no focal neurological deficit was demonstrated.

What is meningism?

Meningism is a sign of irritation of the meninges. It is the triad of:

1 Headache
2 Photophobia
3 Nuchal rigidity. This is the inability to bend the head forward because of rigidity of the neck muscles. If the patient has a full range of motion, even if painful, then by definition nuchal rigidity is absent.

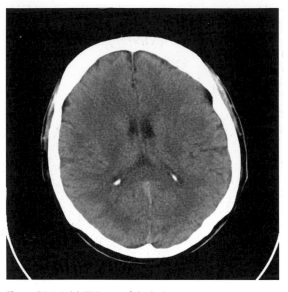

Figure 24.1 Axial CT image of the brain.

What imaging investigation should you request in the first instance?

A CT study of the brain should be requested urgently. This is the most sensitive investigation in the acute phase for identifying haemorrhage. It is readily available, can be performed quickly and will identify any intracerebral mass lesions.

> Mr Black's head CT was reported as 'No intracranial haemorrhage seen (Fig. 24.1). No focal cerebral lesions. I note there is dilatation of the temporal horns of the lateral ventricles, but the remainder of the CSF spaces are normal.'

What proportion of patients with subarachnoid haemorrhage have a normal CT?

When performed within the first 24 hours, CT will demonstrate haemorrhage in around 95% of cases. After the first day, the sensitivity of CT falls.

What is the significance of the temporal horn dilatation?

This is an indirect sign of subarachnoid haemorrhage (SAH) and may be seen even in the absence of high density blood.

What immediate further investigation does Mr Black require?

A lumbar puncture should be performed in the first instance. When the diagnosis of SAH is suspected, at least three tubes of CSF should be collected and labelled in order. The presence of an elevated number of red blood cells, seen equally in all samples, indicates an SAH. A traumatic tap is the more likely cause if the number of red blood cells decreases with each bottle. The CSF sample can also be examined for xanthochromia or with spectrophotometry to detect bilirubin. However, this latter feature takes up to 12 hours as the red blood cells break down and the haem metabolized to bilirubin.

> The CSF samples confirm that Simon has had an SAH.

What are the causes of subarachnoid haemorrhage?

By far the most common cause of an SAH is a leak or rupture of a saccular or 'berry' cerebral aneurysm, accounting for some 80% of cases. Other causes are listed in Box 24.1.

What further investigations should be performed?

The next step is to try to determine the cause of the SAH (i.e. to try and find an underlying vascular abnormality). In recent years, CT angiography has replaced conventional angiography as the initial investigation when looking for aneurysms or vascular malformations.

> However, before this can be performed, Simon becomes unresponsive and has a generalized seizure.

How would you manage this?

- Ensure the airway is maintained safely
- Oxygen
- Monitor and support circulation
- Anti-epileptic agents as required

Box 24.1 Causes of subarachnoid haemorrhage (SAH)

- Cerebral 'berry' aneurysms (80–85% of cases)
- Arteriovenous malformation
- Haemorrhage of brain tumours
- Cocaine use
- Sickle cell anaemia, usually in children
- Anticoagulation therapy
- Trauma

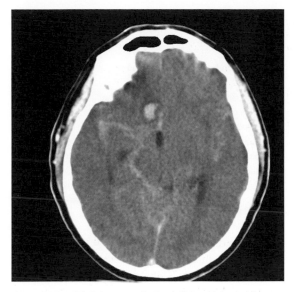

Figure 24.2 Axial CT image at the level of the third ventricle.

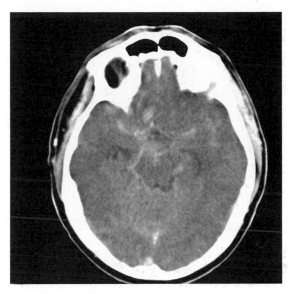

Figure 24.3 Axial CT image at the level of the midbrain.

What investigation does Mr Black require immediately?

A repeat CT examination of the head with angiography.

Once stabilized, Mr Black underwent a CT of the head and CT angiography before being transferred to a high dependency unit.

What do these images show?

The unenhanced axial CT images in Figs 24.2 and 24.3 show that many of the CSF spaces contain high density material. This represents acute SAH in the basal cisterns and right sylvian fissure, as well as an acute parenchymal haematoma in the postero-medial aspect of the right frontal lobe. The temporal horns of the lateral ventricles are slightly dilated, indicating hydrocephalus.

What risk factors are associated with cerebral aneurysm rupture?

- Smoking
- Hypertension
- Alcohol misuse
- Bleeding disorders
- Post-menopause
- Pregnancy

The probability of rupture also depends on the size of the aneurysm. Those measuring less than 5 mm in diameter have a low chance of rupture, of the order of 1% per year. Conversely, two-fifths of those aneurysms measuring 6–10 mm present following rupture.

Are there any other conditions that are associated with cerebral aneurysms?

- Polycystic kidneys
- Coarctation of the aorta
- Ehlers–Danlos syndrome
- Genetic link – close relations appear to have an increased risk of SAH

What do these images show?

There is a 7-mm long aneurysm arising from the anterior communicating artery which is directed inferiorly. The aneurysm can be seen to have a narrow neck (Figs 24.4 and 24.5).

Is this a common site for a cerebral aneurysm?

Yes, aneurysms tend to form at junctions of the major arteries, principally:

- Junction of the posterior communicating artery with the internal carotid artery
- Junction of the anterior communicating artery with the anterior cerebral artery
- Bifurcation of the middle cerebral artery
- Apex of the basilar artery

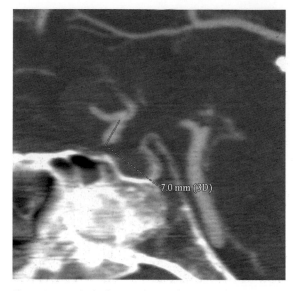

Figure 24.4 Sagittal reformatted image from a CT angiogram.

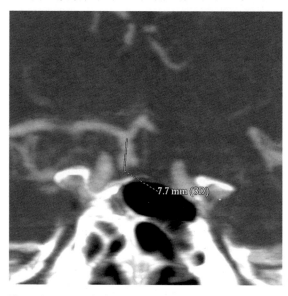

Figure 24.5 Coronal reformatted image from a CT angiogram.

Approximately 1 in 7 patients will have more than one aneurysm.

How is the extent and severity of subarachnoid haemorrhage classified?

There are two clinical classifications in common usage: Hunt and Hess and the World Federation of Neurological Surgeons (WFNS) systems. Both of these grading systems have been shown to correlate well with patient

---

> **Box 24.2 Classifications used in subarachnoid haemorrhage**
>
> **Hunt and Hess classification**
> * Grade 1 – Asymptomatic or mild headache
> * Grade 2 – Moderate to severe headache, nuchal rigidity, with no neurological deficit other than possible cranial nerve palsy
> * Grade 3 – Mild alteration in mental status (confusion, lethargy) with a mild focal neurological deficit
> * Grade 4 – Stupor and/or hemiparesis
> * Grade 5 – Comatose and/or decerebrate rigidity
>
> **World Federation of Neurosurgeons**
> * Grade 1 – Glasgow Coma Score (GCS) 15 without any motor deficit
> * Grade 2 – GCS of 13–14 without any motor deficit
> * Grade 3 – GCS of 13–14 with motor deficit
> * Grade 4 – GCS of 7–12 +/– motor deficit
> * Grade 5 – GCS of 3–6 +/– motor deficit
>
> **Fischer classification (based on CT appearance)**
> * Group 1 – No haemorrhage detected
> * Group 2 – Diffuse deposition of subarachnoid blood. No clots nor layers of blood >1 mm deep
> * Group 3 – Localized clots and/or vertical layers of blood ≥1 mm deep
> * Group 4 – Diffuse or no subarachnoid blood, but intracerebral or intraventricular clots are present

outcome. A third system, the Fischer scale, uses the CT scan appearance and quantification of subarachnoid blood to assess severity. This classification may be used to predict the likelihood of the patient developing symptomatic cerebral vasospasm, a potentially devastating complication in SAH. All of these classifications are useful in determining the optimal management for each patient, but must be used in the context of the patient's overall clinical state (Box 24.2).

What are the priorities in managing patients with SAH?

There are several strands to this which can be categorized in to supportive measures, treatment of the aneurysm to prevent further bleeding and the prevention and management of complications. These are covered in more detail in Box 24.3.

A particular concern is vasospasm, which may develop as a secondary phenomenon following SAH. The spasm may be sufficiently severe to induce an ischaemic

> **Box 24.3 Key points in the management of subarachnoid haemorrhage**
>
> **Supportive measures**
> - Airway management
> - Regular observations
> - Close control of blood pressure
> - Analgesia
> - Nutrition (oral or nasogastic feeding is preferable over parenteral routes)
> - Consider catheterization to monitor fluid balance
>
> **Prevention of re-bleeding**
> - Neurosurgical mangement – clipping of the aneurysm
> - Neuroradiological management – coiling of the aneurysm
>
> **Prevention and management of complications**
> - Neurological complications:
>   - vasospasm (see main text)
>   - hydrocephalus
> - Cardiac complications
> - Electrolyte disturbances
> - Respiratory complications, e.g. pneumonia or pulmonary oedema
> - Deep venous thrombosis prophylaxis

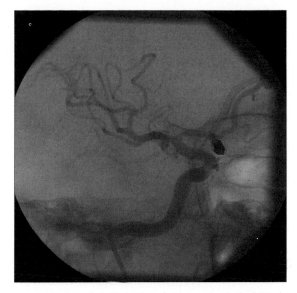

Figure 24.6 Post-procedural right Internal carotid angiogram shows the aneurysm completely occluded by detachable platinum coils.

What treatment options are available for Mr Black's aneurysm?

Cerebral aneurysms may be treated by a surgical approach or radiological approach. Surgery essentially involves placing a clip across the neck of the aneurysm, whereas an endovascular approach involves the placement of coils within the aneurysm sac to induce thrombosis. Each has its place in management and the clinical decision will depend upon the clinical state of the patient; size, number and morphology of the aneurysms; and comorbidities.

Simon underwent endovascular treatment of his cerebral aneurysm which proved to be successful, as can be seen in Fig. 24.6. He made a slow recovery and was left with residual neurological deficits.

cerebrovascular event, thus compounding the clinical problem. In order to try to prevent this occurring, several strategies are employed:

- *Nimodipine:* calcium-channel blocker that appears to reduce spasm and improve survival
- *Hydration:* ensure the patient is well hydrated
- *Blood pressure control:* ensure that hypotension is avoided as this could exacerbate the situation

CASE REVIEW

Simon Black, a 30-year-old nurse, presented to the accident and emergency department with a thunderclap headache. The doctor found evidence of meningism on examination and immediately requested a CT of the head. Although no blood was seen on the initial study, dilatation of the temporal horns of the lateral ventricles was noted and Mr Black proceeded to have a lumbar puncture which confirmed the clinical suspicion of SAH.

Before further investigations could be performed, Simon deteriorated clinically and had a generalized seizure.

A repeat CT study demonstrated the presence of SAH; a CT angiogram demonstrated a 7-mm saccular aneurysm arising from the anterior communicating artery and directed inferiorly.

The aneurysm was treated by the neuroradiologist inserting coils in to the aneurysm sac via an endovascular approach. This was successful and Simon was managed according to standard practice on the wards. He has made a slow recovery but has regained many of his normal functions.

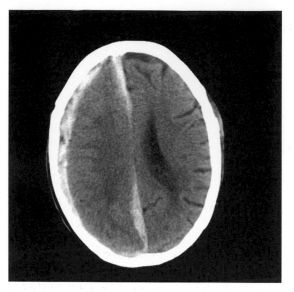

Figure 24.7 Subdural haemorrhage. An unenhanced axial CT shows an acute right convexity subdural haematoma with parafalcine extension. Mass effect effaces the cortical sulci on the right and causes subfalcine herniation ('midline shift') to the left.

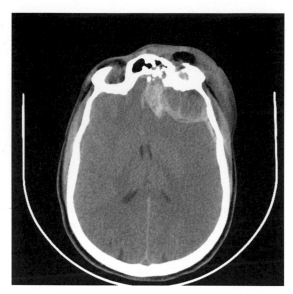

Figure 24.8 Extradural haemorrhage. An unenhanced axial CT shows an acute extradural haematoma overlying the left frontal lobe. The presence of low attenuation within the haematoma ('swirl sign') indicates active bleeding. There is a fracture through the left frontal sinus, which contains haemorrhage, and swelling in the left frontal scalp.

KEY POINTS

- Thunderclap headache is not specific, but is associated with a number of medical emergencies
- Meningism is the triad of headache, photophobia and nuchal rigidity
- If there is any clinical concern, a CT head should be performed as a matter of urgency
- A normal CT does not exclude SAH
- A lumbar puncture is mandatory if the CT does not demonstrate blood
- The cause of SAH is most commonly a saccular aneurysm
- CT angiography is used to identify aneurysms and plan therapy

- Staging classifications may be used to predict vasospasm and clinical outcome
- Cerebral aneurysms may be treated surgically or radiologically
- The management of SAH involves many disciplines, each of which is key to optimizing the outcome
- It is important to be able to differentiate SAH from subdural haemorrhage and extradural haemorrhage, for which the cause and treatment are vastly different. Examples of these can be seen in Figs 24.7 and 24.8, respectively.

Case 25 A 50-year-old woman with a cough

Mrs Amin, a 50-year-old Somalian refugee, presents to her local accident and emergency department. Her English is poor, but she manages to tell you that she has had a cough and felt generally unwell for a month or so. She finds it difficult to explain her symptoms to you.

What would you do now?

It is imperative that you gain as full a clinical history as possible. In order to do so, an interpreter should be engaged to help find out the full history. When doing so, it is often helpful to write down your questions in order to avoid confusion and so that nothing is omitted.

What are the most important points to cover in the clinical history?

Presenting complaint

- Is the cough productive?
- Haemoptysis?
- Chest pain?
- Short of breath?
- Weight loss?
- Night sweats?

Past medical history

- Previous similar episodes?
- HIV? This is very common in sub-Saharan Africa

Medication and allergies
Social history

- Home circumstances
- Smoking, alcohol and recreational drugs
- Foreign travel

Radiology: Clinical Cases Uncovered. By A. S. Shaw, E. M. Godfrey, A. Singh and T. F. Massoud. Published 2009 by Blackwell Publishing. ISBN 978-1-4051-8474-8.

It transpires that Mrs Amin came to the UK 6 months ago as a refugee from Somalia. She has been feeling unwell for over 3 months but has felt particularly poorly in the last 6 weeks. She complains of a cough, occasionally productive of sputum, which is associated with some chest pain. Recently she has also noticed blood mixed with this phlegm on occasion. Not feeling the urge to eat, she says that her clothes are now too loose for her. Recently, Mrs Amin has woken at night on a number of occasions drenched in sweat. What troubles her most is constant fatigue and generally feeling ill.

Mrs Amin lives in a refugee hostel and shares a room with her husband, another Somalian refugee. Her only son also lives in the same hostel. She smokes 15 cigarettes a day and confesses to drinking half a bottle of spirits a week. She denies using intravenous recreational drugs but admits to regularly smoking marijuana.

On examination Mrs Amin appears slightly cachectic, but her cardiorespiratory system appears to be normal.

What are the most likely differential diagnoses in this case?

The clinical features indicate the presence of a progressive pathological process within the lungs, with weight loss and haemoptysis of particular concern. Mrs Amin's history suggests risk factors for bronchogenic malignancy (smoking), infection (poor housing, refugee from a region with endemic tuberculosis (TB) and highly prevalent HIV). The presence of night sweats also raises the possibility of lymphoma, again seen more commonly in patients with HIV.

What initial investigations would you request?

- Full blood count – to look for anaemia or signs of infection
- Urea and electrolytes – to check renal function

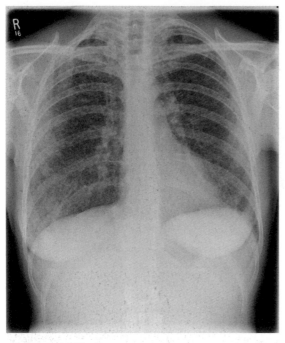

Figure 25.1 PA chest X-ray.

- C-reactive protein (CRP) or erythrocyte sedimentation rate – markers of inflammation
- Chest X-ray (Fig. 25.1)

What does Mrs Amin's chest X-ray show?

The heart size is within normal limits. The mediastinal contours are normal with no evidence of hilar or mediastinal lymphadenopathy. The lungs are of normal volume, but there are widespread nodular deposits throughout both hemithoraces. The nodules are all very small, measuring just a few millimetres across (often termed 'miliary'). There is no pleural effusion.

What is the differential diagnosis for miliary (≤2 mm) nodules throughout both lungs?

- Malignancy:
  - breast
  - thyroid
- Infection:
  - tuberculosis
  - fungal
- Other:
  - sarcoidosis
  - acute extrinsic allergic alveolitis

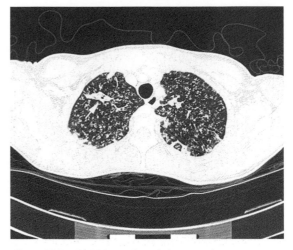

Figure 25.2 Axial CT image through the upper thorax.

What are the most likely diagnoses?

In light of the history and chest X-ray appearances, the main differential diagnoses are disseminated malignancy or TB.

The blood tests revealed Mrs Amin to be anaemic with a haemoglobin count of 10.4 g/dL, with a raised white cell count of 14 × 10⁹/L. The inflammatory markers were found to be elevated with the CRP 60 mg/L. Mrs Amin was referred to the respiratory team for further management.

What would you do now?

1 Establish what the disease process is:
  - Sputum microscopy and culture
  - Bronchoscopy if this is inconclusive
2 Establish the extent of disease (malignant or infective):
  - CT of the chest, abdomen and pelvis
3 Isolate the patient:
  - Until the diagnosis of TB has been excluded

Mrs Amin was referred for CT examination of the chest, abdomen and pelvis.

What do the thoracic images show?

There are widespread miliary nodules with generalized and symmetrical involvement of both lungs with no zonal or lobar predominance (Figs 25.2–25.4). In the lung apices, there are a few areas of more confluent consolidation, with a small area of cavitation present within

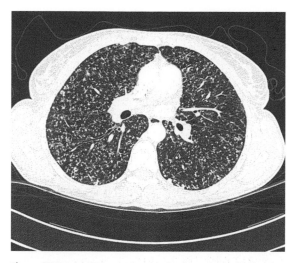

Figure 25.3 Axial CT image through the thorax at the level of the main pulmonary artery.

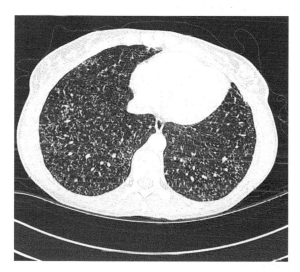

Figure 25.4 Axial CT image through the lower thorax.

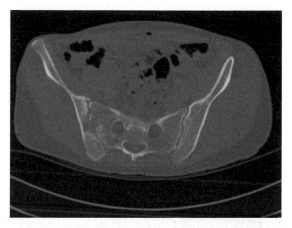

Figure 25.5 Axial CT image through the pelvis on bone windows.

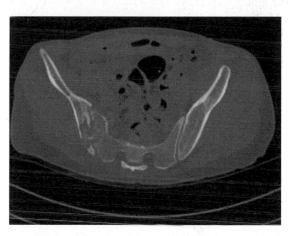

Figure 25.6 Axial CT image through the pelvis on bone windows.

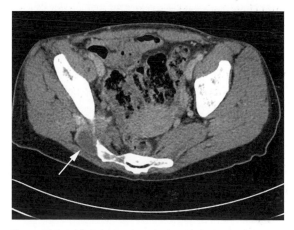

Figure 25.7 Axial CT image through the pelvis on soft tissue windows.

the right upper lobe (Fig. 25.2). No hilar, mediastinal or axillary lymphadenopathy was seen. There is no pleural effusion.

What abnormalities can be seen on the pelvic images?

There is bony destruction involving the right sacrum and ilium on either side of the right sacroiliac joint, hence the process is centred upon the sacroiliac joint (Figs 25.5–25.7). The sclerotic focus of bone within the lytic area is

Box 25.1 Miliary tuberculosis

- Rare but feared complication of both primary and post primary TB
- Massive haematogenous dissemination of the disease which can occur any time following the primary infection
- 2–3% of all TB infections
- Myriad of 2–3 mm granulomatous foci uniformly distributed and of equal size
- Usually recognizable 6 weeks post haematogenous dissemination
- Can affect a number of organs: lymph nodes, liver, spleen, bones, kidneys, adrenal glands, prostate, testes, fallopian tubes, endometrium, brain and meninges
- Miliary TB does not leave residual calcification and clears rapidly with appropriate therapy

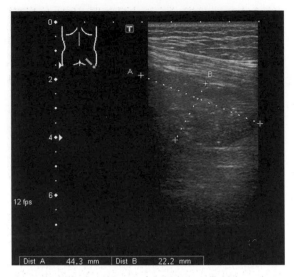

Figure 25.8 Ultrasound image of the right sacroiliac joint region confirming the presence of a 4.4 × 2.2 cm abscess.

devascularized and is called the sequestrum. On the lower image on soft tissue windows, a discrete fluid collection can be seen at the inferior aspect of the joint (Fig. 25.7, arrow). The imaging features are those of right-sided septic sacroiliitis.

What is the unifying diagnosis?
Disseminated TB resulting in miliary nodules throughout the lungs (Box 25.1), sacroiliitis and an abscess.

Can you start therapy based on these characteristic appearances?
No, the treatment for TB is lengthy and carries its own risks. More importantly, it is vital to obtain microbiological samples to determine whether there is any drug resistance.

What are the common investigations used to confirm a diagnosis of TB in the hospital setting?
- Multiple sputum samples for microscopy, culture and sensitivity for acid-fast bacilli (AFB)
- AFB resist acid–alcohol decolorization under Ziehl–Neelsen staining and are cultured with prolonged incubation on Lowenstein–Jensen medium
- More rapid diagnosis may be achieved with polymerase chain reaction (PCR) technology

- Bronchoscopy with biopsy and/or bronchoalveolar lavage
- Histology will show caseating granulomas

A diagnosis of TB was confirmed by both microbiology and histology following bronchoscopy. The presumed tuberculous abscess seen at the right sacroiliac joint was further assessed with ultrasound (Fig. 25.8). This was drained under ultrasound guidance and specimens later confirmed the presence of AFB.

What would be a typical treatment for TB?
- Initial phase (2 months, four drugs):
  - rifampicin
  - isoniazid (with pyridoxine, to help avoid side-effects)
  - pyrazinamide
  - ethambutol (if resistance possible)
- Continuation phase (4 months, two drugs):
  - rifampicin
  - isoniazid
  - ethambutol if resistance suspected

What other important points need to be considered?
- Patient:
  - counselling for HIV testing

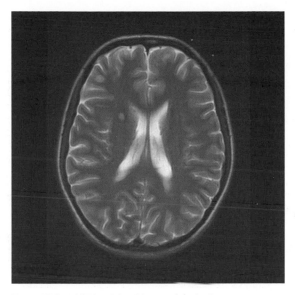

Figure 25.9 Axial T2-weighted image of the brain.

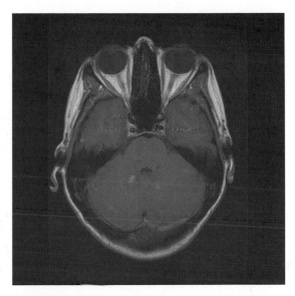

Figure 25.10 Axial T1-weighted image of the brain following intravenous gadolinium.

○ counselling of the patient with particular reference to the prolonged treatment, strict adherence to treatment and its side-effects
• Public health:
  ○ notification to the consultant in communicable disease control
  ○ contact tracing and screening
  ○ measures to prevent spread to other individuals in the community and in her home

Mrs Amin was commenced on multiple anti tuberculous agents as per standard protocol and later discharged. She was followed up as an outpatient but there were suspicions that her compliance to the treatment regimen was poor, although she denied this.

Four months later she began complaining of headaches, dizziness, nausea and severe general malaise. She was again admitted to hospital for further investigation and an MRI study of the brain was performed.

The unenhanced T1-weighted images were normal. What do these images show?

The T2-weighted image shows small foci of high signal (Fig. 25.9). On the T1-weighted images there are multiple small enhancing nodules measuring up to 5 mm in both cerebral hemispheres (Figs 25.10–25.12). Some of these lesions have an area of ring enhancement and the

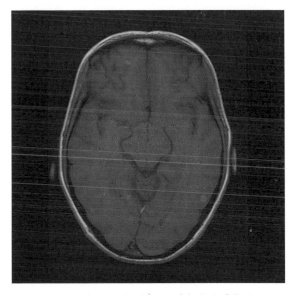

Figure 25.11 Axial T1-weighted image of the brain following intravenous gadolinium.

majority of lesions are located at the grey–white matter interface. There is no midline shift or meningeal enhancement.

What is the likely diagnosis?

The appearances would be consistent with TB involving the brain.

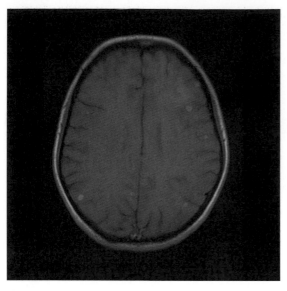

Figure 25.12 Axial T1-weighted image of the brain following intravenous gadolinium.

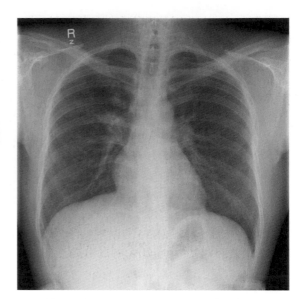

Figure 25.13 Frontal chest X-ray.

Mrs Amin was given therapy as an inpatient initially. Following discharge, she was referred to the local DOTS programme. This is Directly Observed Therapy, which ensures high compliance, improves cure rate and helps to reduce drug resistance; it is a central tool in the global fight against TB.

Following contact tracing, Mrs Amin's husband was screened for infection. Recently, he too had been feeling unwell with a history of lethargy and weight loss.

What do his results show?

The heart size is normal (Fig. 25.13). However, the right hilum appears rather bulky with some ill-defined opacities in the adjacent lung parenchyma. The left hemithorax appears clear and there are no pleural effusions. This is suspicious for tuberculous infection (Box 25.2).

A CT scan of the chest was performed to further assess the abnormalities seen on the chest X-ray.

What abnormalities are seen on these images?

Several small foci of consolidation are seen within the right upper lobe and the apical segment of the right lower lobe (Figs 25.14 and 25.15). In the latter, there is early cavitation seen. These features suggest active TB infection (Box 25.3).

Box 25.2 Features of tuberculosis on chest radiographs

Primary tuberculosis
- Pneumonia mimicking community-acquired pneumonia
- Any lobe
- Ipsilateral hilar/mediastinal node enlargement
- Associated pleural effusions in younger patients
- Following resolution, one-third develop a residual well-defined rounded or linear opacity +/– calcification = Ghon focus
- Ghon focus + ipsilateral lymph node calcification = Ranke Complex
- Ghon focus or Ranke Complex reflects a previous primary TB infection but not disease activity

Post primary tuberculosis
- Most develop nodular and linear opacities in the apico-posterior segment of the upper lobe and/or apical segment of the lower lobe
- Unilateral or bilateral
- Cavitation
- Fibrosis
- Pleural thickening
- Volume loss
- Pleural effusion/empyema

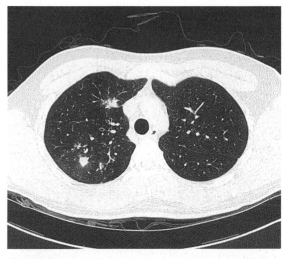

Figure 25.14 Axial CT image of the upper thorax.

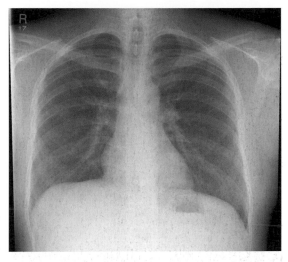

Figure 25.16 Frontal chest X-ray.

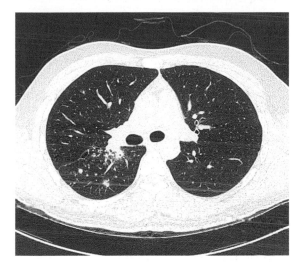

Figure 25.15 Axial CT image through the thorax at the level of the main pulmonary artery.

Box 25.3 CT features indicating active tuberculous disease

- Centrilobular nodules or 'tree in bud' branching structures
- Ground glass opacities
- Consolidation
- Cavitation
- Miliary nodules
- Interlobular septal thickening
- Pleural or pericardial effusion
- Lymph nodes with low attenuation centres and peripheral rim enhancement

---

Biopsies confirmed AFB and Mr Amin was also commenced on anti-TB chemotherapy and was followed closely in clinic. Figure 25.16 shows a follow-up chest X-ray performed 4 months later.

How would you interpret this?

The right hilar lymphadenopathy has resolved, with a corresponding improvement in the appearances of the right lung. These features indicate a good response to anti-TB therapy.

Six months later, Mr and Mrs Amin's son, Desmond, presented with severe right-sided lower back pain. He had been screened for TB following his parents' illness and nothing untoward had been found. On examination, he appeared to have some loss of sensation and was referred for an MRI study of his whole spine.

What does the MRI study show?

There is a pathological compressive fracture of the C3 vertebral body with retropulsion of bone posteriorly causing some compromise to the bony canal. There is also marrow replacement at this level and an associated soft tissue component anteriorly (Figs 25.17–25.19).

On the lower images, one can see a posterior extradural large soft tissue mass at the level of T11 with compromise of the spinal canal. On the axial images, one can see

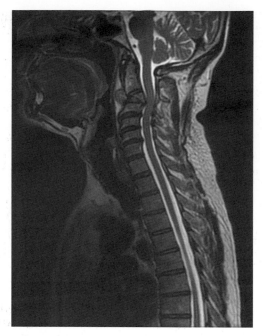

Figure 25.17 Sagittal T2-weighted image of the cervico-thoracic spine.

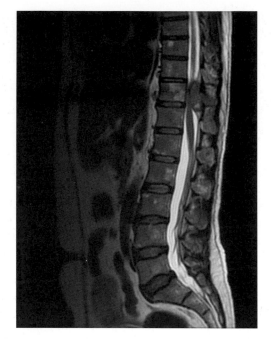

Figure 25.18 Sagittal T2-weighted image of the thoraco-lumbar spine.

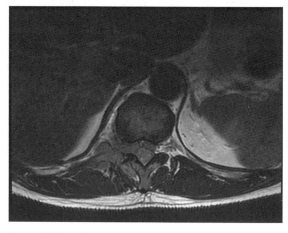

Figure 25.19 Axial T2-weighted image through the lower thoracic spine.

> ### Box 25.4 MRI appearances of tuberculous infections involving the spine
>
> - MRI is the preferred technique to diagnose infective disorders of the spine
> - Early signs are low signal throughout the disc and adjacent parts of the vertebral body on T1-weighted images with high signal on T2-weighted images
> - Loss of vertebral end plate margins and vertebral collapse
> - Paraspinal and epidural abscesses
> - Diffuse enhancement of infected area on administration of intravenous gadolinium. NB Pus will not enhance
> - In spinal TB the most common site affected is the thoraco-lumbar junction

the cord being displaced to the left by the mass which involves the vertebral body and extends in to the neural foramen. These features are all consistent with spinal TB infection (Box 25.4).

Desmond underwent a CT-guided biopsy. The histopathology report described 'granulomas cuffed by lymphocytes, rare plasma cells and containing multinucleate giant cells. The findings are typical of Mycobacterium infection.' Desmond was also commenced on multiagent anti-TB therapy and made a good recovery.

CASE REVIEW

Mrs Amin, a 50-year-old Somalian who had recently come to the UK presented with a 3-month history of cough, malaise, night sweats, weight loss and haemoptysis. Her chest X-ray and high resolution CT indicated the high possibility of disseminated tuberculous infection. This was confirmed on sputum culture and histology following a bronchoscopic biopsy. Axial CT of the chest, abdomen and pelvis also identified abnormalities in the right sacroiliac joint with an associated abscess. Ultrasound-guided drainage confirmed this also was the focus of TB infection. Mrs Amin was commenced on anti-TB therapy but was poorly compliant, and as a consequence her condition was further complicated by cerebral infection.

Following contact tracing her husband, Mr Amin, was screened for TB. Chest X-rays and subsequent CT findings were consistent with active pulmonary TB which was confirmed on biopsy. He was compliant with therapy and made a good recovery.

Despite initial screening, Mr and Mrs Amin's son Desmond presented 6 months later with severe back pain and loss of sensation. Imaging the whole spine revealed multiple foci of infection with bony destruction and displacement of the spinal cord. He too made a good recovery following treatment.

KEY POINTS

- A high level of suspicion should be held in appropriate patient groups
- A thorough social history is essential when investigating a patient suspected of having TB
- Microbiological or histopathological confirmation is required before commencing treatment
- Notification to the consultant in communicable diseases is a legal requirement
- Contact tracing and screening with appropriate counselling are essential
- Adherence to treatment schedule is paramount and the patient should be monitored closely
- Failure of compliance can lead to relapse and drug resistance

- DOTS should be considered in patients with poor compliance
- A chest X-ray is not diagnostic of pulmonary TB but features such as cavitation, fibrosis, calcification and pleural thickening in the upper zones with hilar lymphadenopathy should greatly raise the suspicion on the background of a suggestive history
- CT is recommended where plain radiography is normal or equivocal where there is a suspicion of TB or its complications
- Miliary TB is a very serious and potentially life-threatening complication that requires early detection and aggressive treatment
- MRI is the preferred modality when assessing infections involving the brain and spine

MCQs

For each situation, choose the single option you feel is most correct.

---

1 *A 43-year-old lady presents with colicky right upper quadrant pain which is exacerbated by eating fatty foods.*

Which of the following radiological investigations should you request?
a. Chest X-ray
b. Abdominal ultrasound
c. Abdominal CT
d. Abdominal X-ray
e. Magnetic resonance cholangiopancreatography (MRCP)

---

2 *True pulmonary cysts are a feature of:*

a. Langerhans cell histiocytosis
b. Sarcoidosis
c. Emphysema
d. Fibrosing alveolitis
e. Bronchiectasis

---

3 *A 75-year-old lady with severe chronic obstructive pulmonary disease (COPD) presents with acute breathlessness. The chest X-ray shows there is no focal consolidation. She is afebrile, but D-dimers are markedly elevated.*

Which of the following investigations should you request next?

Radiology: Clinical Cases Uncovered. By A. S. Shaw, E. M. Godfrey, A. Singh and T. F. Massoud. Published 2009 by Blackwell Publishing. ISBN 978-1-4051-8474-8.

a. Pulmonary angiography
b. Ventilation–perfusion (V/Q) scan
c. High resolution CT thorax
d. CT pulmonary angiography
e. Lateral chest X-ray

---

4 *Which of the following tumours most commonly gives sclerotic bone metastases?*

a. Lung
b. Renal
c. Prostate
d. Ovary
e. Thyroid

---

5 *In which of the following CNS diseases do lesions typically exhibit uniform enhancement following intravenous contrast medium?*

a. Toxoplasmosis
b. Metastasis
c. Glioblastoma multiforme
d. Tuberculosis
e. Lymphoma

---

6 *Which of the following features of MRI suggest that lesions are caused by ischaemia rather than multiple sclerosis?*

a. Ovoid high signal foci on T2-weighted images
b. Involvement of the corpus callosum
c. Uniform enhancement following administration of intravenous gadolinium
d. Perivenular distribution (perpendicular to ventricles)
e. Involvement of the thalamus

7 *Which of the following conditions is not associated with an increased risk of developing malignancy?*

a. Pseudomembranous colitis
b. Ulcerative colitis
c. Coeliac disease
d. Primary sclerosing cholangitis
e. Crohn's colitis

8 *The most common solid abdominal tumour of childhood is:*

a. Hepatoblastoma
b. Neuroblastoma
c. Wilms' tumour
d. Hepatocellular carcinoma
e. Teratoma

9 *Which of the following returns a high signal on T1-weighted MRI?*

a. Cerebrospinal fluid
b. Cortical bone
c. Haemosiderin
d. Methaemoglobin
e. Flowing blood

10 *Which of the following is not a feature of cystic fibrosis?*

a. Bronchiectasis
b. Pancreatitis
c. Cirrhosis
d. Infertility
e. Diabetes insipidus

11 *Which of the following is not a contraindication to a contrast-enhanced MRI of the liver?*

a. Total hip replacement 3 months ago
b. Intra-ocular metallic foreign body
c. Acute renal failure
d. Cardiac pacemaker
e. Cochlear implant

12 *Breast cancer screening of standard risk patients:*

a. Is offered to all women over 40 years of age in the UK
b. Comprises triple assessment with examination, ultrasound and mammography
c. Comprises ultrasound and mammography alone
d. Comprises mammography alone on a 3-yearly basis
e. Has made little impact on mortality from breast cancer

13 *With respect to tuberculosis infection:*

a. Primary infection has a predilection for the lower lobe
b. Pleural effusions are a feature of post-primary infection
c. Imaging appearances are sufficiently specific to commence therapy
d. Non-caseating granulomas on biopsy are diagnostic
e. Miliary disease results in calcified granulomas following therapy

14 *With respect to paediatric imaging, ultrasound is not the initial investigation of choice for:*

a. Suspected appendicitis
b. Suspected intussusception
c. Urinary infection
d. Blunt abdominal trauma
e. Projectile vomiting in infants

15 *With regard to the imaging of a foreign body:*

a. Wood is rarely radio-opaque
b. Glass is rarely radio-opaque
c. An abdominal radiograph should be performed to identify the object
d. Plastic is usually radio-opaque
e. Ultrasound is rarely of value when the lesion is not radio-opaque

16 *Follow-up of patient who had previously undergone an endovascular aortic (EVAR) stent insertion reports 'filling of the aneurysm sac distally because of ineffective seal of the stent graft'.*

What type of endoleak is this?
a. Type I
b. Type II
c. Type III
d. Type IV
e. Type V

17 *With regard to acute pancreatitis:*

a. Ultrasound should always be performed to confirm the diagnosis
b. CT should be performed to look for gallstones
c. MRCP should be performed in the acute phase to look for common bile duct stones
d. The presence of necrosis should prompt early surgical intervention
e. Pseudocysts do not develop within the first 2 weeks of the acute episode

18 *Which of the following is not a 'major feature' of tuberous sclerosis?*

a. Cortical hamartomas
b. Giant cell astrocytoma
c. Cardiac rhabdomyomas
d. Renal angiomyolipomas
e. Hepatic adenomas

19 *With respect to the branches of the aorta:*

a. The left subclavian artery is usually the first branch
b. The right external carotid artery is usually the second branch
c. The coeliac axis gives rise to the common hepatic and splenic arteries
d. The renal arteries arise just above the superior mesenteric artery
e. The aorta bifurcates at the level of S2

20 *On an X-ray of the foot, a 'rounded erosion with a sclerotic margin and overhanging edge' is seen.*

The most likely diagnosis is:
a. Rheumatoid arthritis
b. Gout
c. Psoriatic arthritis
d. Calcium pyrophosphate arthropathy
e. Osteoarthritis

21 *Which of the following techniques is not helpful in the evaluation of patients with multiple myeloma?*

a. Skeletal survey
b. Bone scintigraphy
c. Positron emission tomography (PET) study
d. Computed tomography
e. Magnetic resonance imaging

22 *A 67-year-old man presents to the accident and emergency department with severe colicky left loin pain and microscopic haematuria.*

Which of the following radiological investigations should you request?
a. Abdominal X-ray
b. Magnetic resonance urography
c. Ultrasound of the renal tract
d. CT of the abdomen and pelvis
e. Intravenous urogram

23 *An abdominal radiograph is reported as showing 'Rigler's sign'.*

What is the most likely diagnosis?
a. Acute pancreatitis
b. Small bowel obstruction
c. Large bowel obstruction
d. Ulcerative colitis
e. Bowel perforation

24 *A patient with known sarcoidosis has bilateral hilar lymphadenopathy but his lungs are clear.*

What stage sarcoid is this?
a. Stage 0
b. Stage I
c. Stage II
d. Stage III
e. Stage IV

25 *A CT report on a patient with metastatic colon cancer reports that they have had a partial response by RECIST criteria.*

What does this mean?
a. All of the lesions are smaller
b. Some of the lesions are no longer visible.
c. The sum of the diameters of the metastases has reduced by 30%
d. The sum of the diameters of the metastases has reduced by 50%
e. The cross-sectional area of the metastases has reduced by 70%

26 *Pulmonary fibrosis predominantly involving the lower lobes is a feature of:*

a. Sarcoidosis
b. Fibrosing alveolitis
c. Tuberculosis
d. Radiotherapy
e. Chronic extrinsic allergic alveolitis

27 *With regard to primary pneumothorax:*

a. An expiratory chest X-ray should be performed to assess the size
b. A chest X-ray is essential in all cases prior to treatment
c. An intercostal chest drain should be used initially to maximize drainage
d. The term 'primary pneumothorax' refers to a patient's first presentation
e. A 2-cm rim of air equates to a 50% pneumothorax

28 *Which of the following hepatic lesions never enhances in the arterial phase of imaging (CT or MRI)?*

a. Hepatic cyst
b. Haemangioma
c. Adenoma
d. Fibrous nodular hyperplasia
e. Hepatocellular carcinoma

29 *Crohn's disease:*

a. Involves the rectum in 95% of cases
b. Involves the colon in continuity
c. May result in a toxic megacolon
d. Is associated with struvite urinary calculi
e. Results in a 'lead-pipe' appearance in the chronic phase

30 *Regarding the pulmonary complications of recreational drug use, which of the following statements is false?*

a. Cocaine can cause pulmonary haemorrhage
b. Marijuana can result in early onset emphysema
c. Opiates can result in pulmonary fibrosis
d. Amphetamines can cause pulmonary oedema
e. Nitrites can cause a lipoid pneumonia

EMQs

1 Period of background radiation

a. 0 days
b. 1 day
c. 3 days
d. 10 days
e. 3 weeks
f. 1 month
g. 2 months
h. 4 months
i. 6 months
j. 10 months
k. 1 year
l. 1.8 years
m. 4.5 years
n. 7.5 years
o. 10 years

For each of the investigations listed below choose the equivalent period of background radiation to which the average adult patient would be exposed. Each answer may be chosen once, more than once or not at all.

1. Chest X-ray
2. CT head
3. Abdominal X-ray
4. Bone scintigraphy (^{99m}Tc-MDP)
5. CT abdomen and pelvis

2 Arteries

a. Right subclavian artery
b. Left subclavian artery
c. Right external carotid artery
d. Pulmonary artery
e. Middle cerebral artery
f. Superficial femoral artery
g. Common iliac artery
h. Basilar artery
i. Bronchial artery
j. Renal artery
k. Common femoral artery
l. Posterior cerebral artery
m. Common hepatic artery
n. Popliteal artery
o. Anterior cerebral artery

For each of the following cases, identify which artery is being described. Each answer may be chosen once, more than once or not at all.

1. It is formed by the confluence of the left and right vertebral arteries.
2. This artery runs in the sylvian fissure.
3. This branch of the thoracic aorta supplies the lungs.
4. This is the ideal site of puncture for percutaneous angiography of the lower limbs.
5. It is formed at the level of L4 by the terminal division of the aorta.

Radiology: Clinical Cases Uncovered. By A. S. Shaw, E. M. Godfrey, A. Singh and T. F. Massoud. Published 2009 by Blackwell Publishing. ISBN 978-1-4051-8474-8.

3 Choice of investigations

a. Leg ultrasound
b. Chest X-ray
c. Abdominal X-ray
d. Ventilation–perfusion (V/Q) scan
e. Venogram
f. CT pulmonary angiogram
g. Magnetic resonance cholangiopancreatography (MRCP)
h. Abdominal ultrasound
i. CT abdomen and pelvis
j. Pulmonary angiogram
k. Endoscopic retrograde cholangiopancreatography (ERCP)
l. MRI liver
m. Pelvic ultrasound
n. Hepatobiliary imino-diacetic acid (HIDA) scan
o. Pelvic MRI

For each of the following clinical presentations, which is the most appropriate initial imaging investigation? Each answer may be chosen once, more than once or not at all.

1. Suspected deep vein thrombosis
2. Jaundice
3. Suspected pulmonary embolism in a patient with emphysema
4. Post-menopausal bleeding
5. Suspected leaking abdominal aortic aneurysm

4 Bones

a. Metacarpal
b. Metatarsal
c. Scaphoid
d. Lunate
e. Radius
f. Ulna
g. Humerus
h. Scapula
i. Sternum
j. Zygoma
k. Sacrum
l. Femur
m. Tibia
n. Fibula
o. Calcaneum

The following are bony abnormalities, but to which bone do they refer? Each answer may be chosen once, more than once or not at all.

1. Colles' fracture
2. Kienböck's disease
3. Perthes' disease
4. Smith's fracture
5. Hill–Sachs lesion

5 **Diagnoses**

a. Pulmonary embolism

b. Fibrosing alveolitis

c. Sarcoidosis

d. Miliary tuberculosis

e. Pneumothorax

f. Pneumonia

g. Lung cancer

h. Pulmonary arteriovenous malformation

i. Pulmonary metastases

j. Pericardial effusion

k. Bone metastases

l. Pleural effusion

m. Lymphoma

n. Ruptured hemidiaphragm

o. Left ventricular aneurysm

For each of the following chest X-rays give the likeliest diagnosis. Each answer may be chosen once, more than once or not at all.

1. Figure E5.1

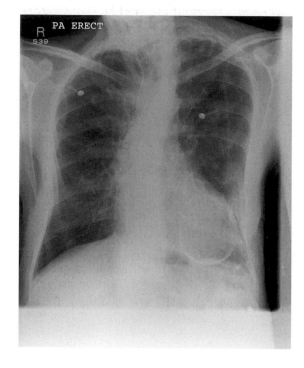

2. Figure E5.2

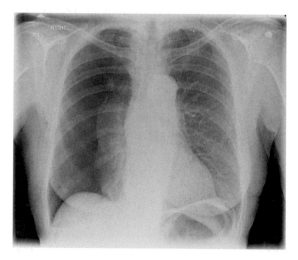

3. Figure E5.3

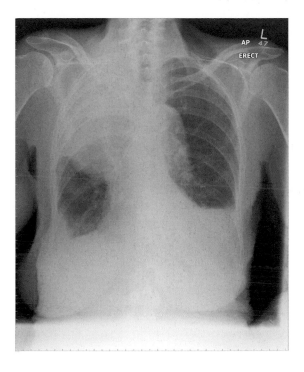

5. Figure E5.5

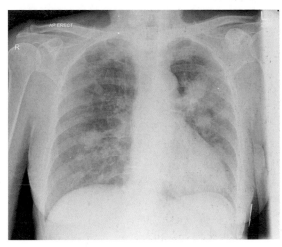

4. Figure E5.4

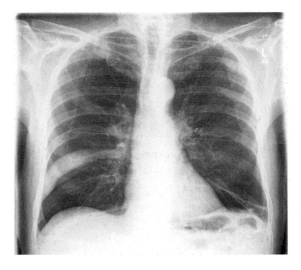

6 Diagnoses

a. Pulmonary embolism
b. Fibrosing alveolitis
c. Sarcoidosis
d. Posterior mediastinal mass
e. Pneumothorax
f. Pneumonia
g. Lung cancer
h. Pulmonary arteriovenous malformation
i. Pulmonary metastases
j. Pneumoperitoneum
k. Bone metastases
l. Pleural effusion
m. Anterior mediastinal mass
n. Ruptured hemidiaphragm
o. Mesothelioma

For each of the following chest X-rays give the likeliest diagnosis. Each answer may be chosen once, more than once or not at all.

1. Figure E6.1

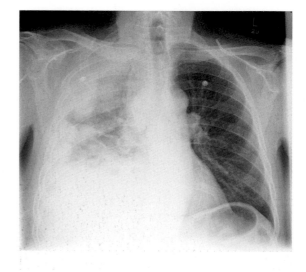

2. Figure E6.2

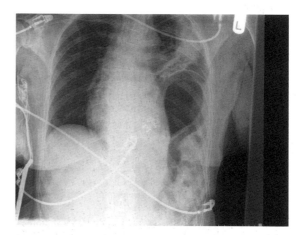

3. Figure E6.3

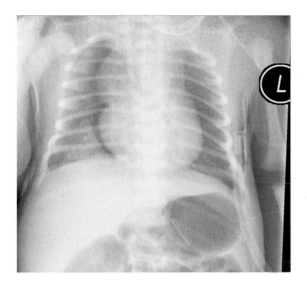

5. Figure E6.5

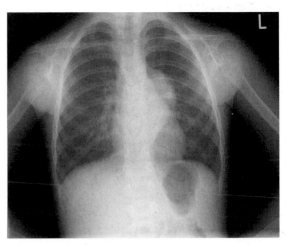

4. Figure E6.4

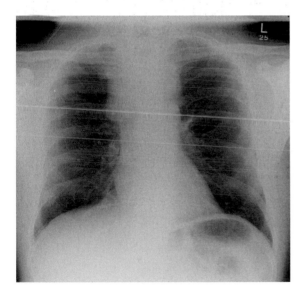

7 Diagnoses

a. Acute pancreatitis

b. Hydatid cyst

c. Inguinal hernia

d. Medullary nephrocalcinosis

e. Gastric volvulus

f. Small bowel obstruction

g. Gallstones

h. Porcelain gallbladder

i. Sigmoid volvulus

j. Chronic pancreatitis

k. Abdominal aortic aneurysm

l. Large bowel obstruction

m. Caecal volvulus

n. Pneumoperitoneum

o. Acute appendicitis

For each of the following abdominal X-rays give the likeliest diagnosis. Each answer may be chosen once, more than once or not at all.

1. Figure E7.1

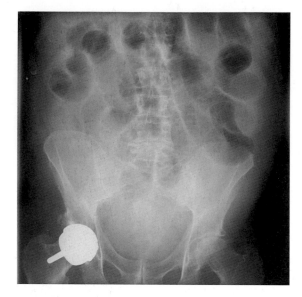

2. Figure E7.2

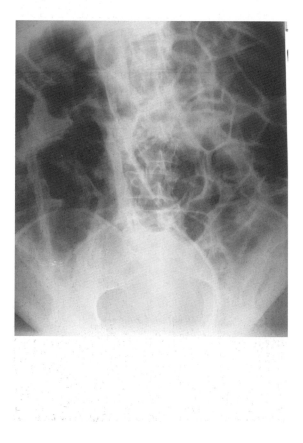

3. Figure E7.3

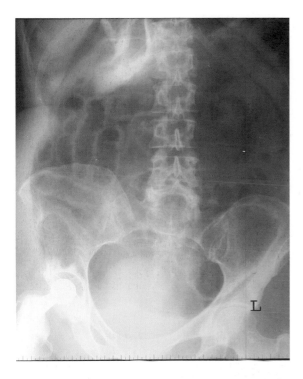

4. Figure E7.4

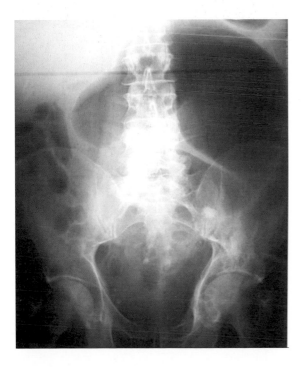

5. Figure E7.5

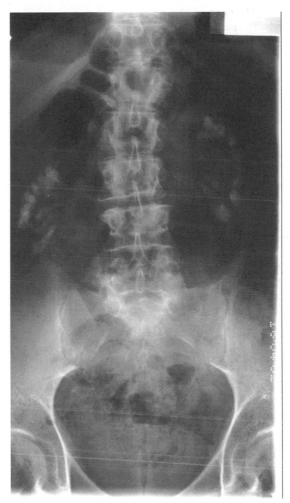

8 Diagnoses

a. Aortic dissection

b. Acute diverticulitis

c. Haemangioma

d. Renal calculi

e. Caecal carcinoma

f. Acute appendicitis

g. Acute pancreatitis

h. Ureteric calculi

i. Renal cell carcinoma

j. Crohn's disease

k. Splenic laceration

l. Transitional cell carcinoma

m. Chronic pancreatitis

n. Lymphoma

o. Splenic metastasis

For each of the following abdominal CT images give the likeliest diagnosis. Each answer may be chosen once, more than once or not at all.

1. Figure E8.1

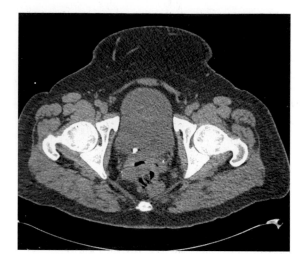

2. Figure E8.2

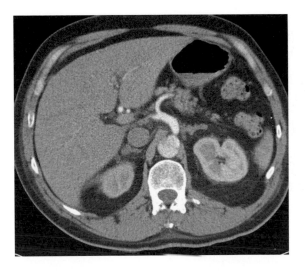

4. Figure E8.4

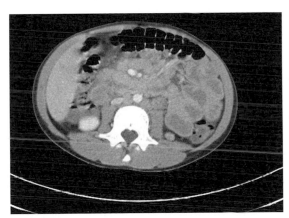

3. Figure E8.3

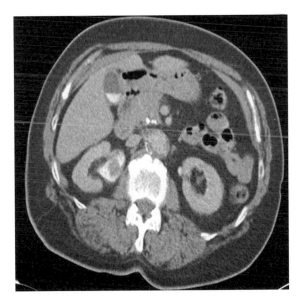

5. Figure E8.5

9 Diagnoses

a. Subarachnoid haemorrhage
b. Pituitary haemorrhage
c. Meningioma
d. Intra-ocular haemorrhage
e. Intracerebral haemorrhage
f. Cerebral metastasis
g. Toxoplasmosis
h. Dermoid tumour
i. Subdural haemorrhage
j. Arteriovenous malformation
k. Ischaemic stroke
l. Extradural haemorrhage
m. Colloid cyst
n. Multiple sclerosis
o. Glioblastoma multiforme

For each of the following head CT images give the likeliest diagnosis. Each answer may be chosen once, more than once or not at all.

1. Figure E9.1

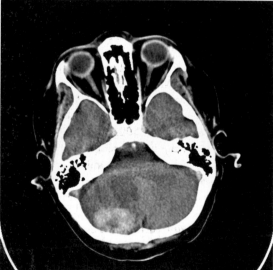

2. Figure E9.2

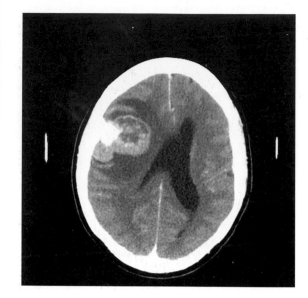

3. Figure E9.3

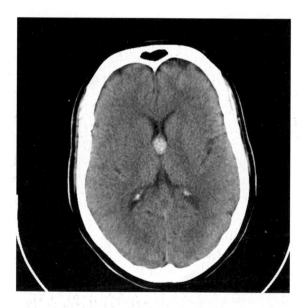

4. Figure E9.4

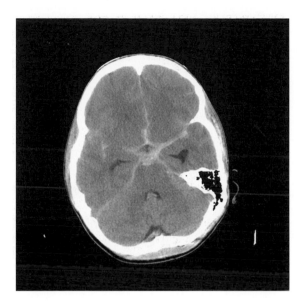

5. Figure E9.5

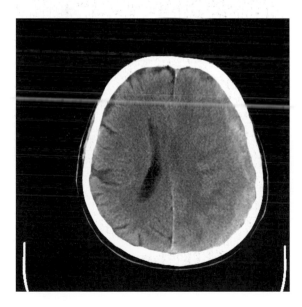

10 Diagnoses

a. Haemangioma
b. Rheumatoid arthritis
c. Angiomyolipoma
d. Lingular lobe consolidation
e. Osteoarthritis
f. Lower lobe consolidation
g. Pneumoperitoneum
h. Small bowel obstruction
i. Hepatocellular carcinoma
j. Middle lobe consolidation
k. Paralytic ileus
l. Renal cell carcinoma
m. Sigmoid volvulus
n. Cyst
o. Gout

The hospital computer system has failed. Your colleague describes each case to you over the telephone. What is the diagnosis? Each answer may be chosen once, more than once or not at all.

1. There is a lesion within the liver seen on MRI. It is of uniform low signal on T1-weighted images, high signal on T2-weighted images and does not enhance following intravenous gadolinium.

2. There is a 4-cm diameter lesion within the right kidney seen on CT. It appears to have a density lower than water but greater than air on the unenhanced images. Following intravenous contrast medium, there is avid enhancement within the lesion but this is rather heterogeneous.

3. On the chest X-ray, there is an opacity in the right lower zone which obscures the right heart border. There is no loss of volume in either lung.

4. On the plain film of the right knee there is loss of joint space, sclerosis of the articular surface, subchondral cyst formation and osteophytes.

5. On the abdominal X-ray, the liver appears less dense than usual and the bladder more dense. It appears as though one can see both sides of the bowel wall in places.

1 *A 56-year-old man with a history of poorly controlled hypertension presents to the accident and emergency department with sudden onset weakness on the left side.*

a. What are the key features in the clinical history? *(3 marks)*
b. What initial investigation(s) would you request? *(2 marks)*
c. The investigations identify an intracranial aneurysm. What are the initial and definitive treatment options? *(3 marks)*
d. What are the potential complications of these treatments? *(2 marks)*

2 *A 24-year-old woman presents to her GP with mildly painful swelling of her right leg. She is 32 weeks pregnant with her second child but is otherwise well and has no other medical history of note.*

a. What are the two likeliest causes for the presenting symptoms? *(2 marks)*
b. What investigation(s) would be of value in this case? Is there any part of your usual practice that you might omit here? *(2 marks)*
c. The results are normal, but 1 week later the patient presents to the accident and emergency department with acute shortness of breath. What diagnosis do you need to exclude? *(1 mark)*
d. How might you investigate the patient radiologically? Give your reasons *(5 marks)*

3 *A 48-year-old man presents to the respiratory team with progressive breathlessness. On examination there are crackles bilaterally. You suspect that the patient may have interstitial lung disease.*

a. What are the key points to elucidate in the clinical history? *(4 marks)*
b. What pattern would you expect to find on pulmonary function tests? *(1 mark)*
c. What are the key features that can be seen on the high resolution CT images (Figures S3.1–S3.4)? *(4 marks)*
d. What is the most likely diagnosis? *(1 mark)*

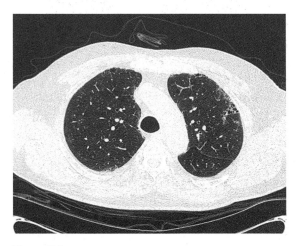

Figure S3.1

Radiology: Clinical Cases Uncovered. By A. S. Shaw, E. M. Godfrey, A. Singh and T. F. Massoud. Published 2009 by Blackwell Publishing. ISBN 978-1-4051-8474-8.

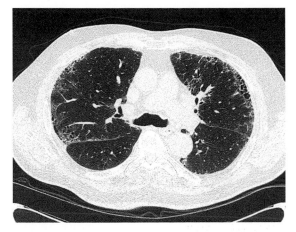

Figure S3.2

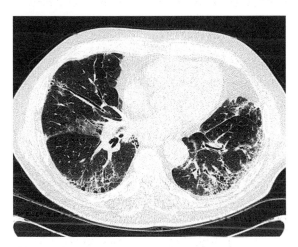

Figure S3.3

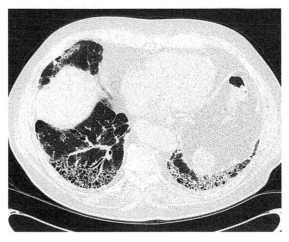

Figure S3.4

4 *A 53-year-old man, well known to his GP with a long history of low back pain, presents once again with similar symptoms. He has had a previous X-ray showing degenerative disc changes 6 years earlier.*

a. He asks to be referred for another X-ray. What is your response? *(2 marks)*
b. What is the approximate equivalent period of background radiation for a lateral X-ray of the lumbar spine? *(1 mark)*
c. What features should raise suspicions in patients with chronic lumbar pain? *(5 marks)*
d. What would you request if these were present? *(2 marks)*

5 *A previously healthy 61-year-old woman presents with a 3-week history of altered bowel habit and rectal bleeding. She refuses to undergo a colonoscopy.*

a. What other options are available to you? *(3 marks)*
b. What are the pros and cons of each investigation? *(6 marks)*
c. Which would you recommend to her? *(1 mark)*

6 *A 45-year-old woman presents to the accident and emergency department with severe central abdominal pain. She has markedly elevated amylase levels.*

a. What imaging investigations should you request to confirm the diagnosis? *(1 mark)*
b. What are the indications for imaging in the acute phase? *(2 marks)*
c. What are the common causes of acute pancreatitis? *(3 marks)*
d. The clinical history provides no clues to the aetiology. What imaging investigations might help and why? *(4 marks)*

7 *A 47-year-old man with chronic hepatitis B infection is referred to you for surveillance.*

a. What is the purpose of the surveillance and how would you carry this out? *(2 marks)*
b. The patient is to undergo a liver biopsy. What does this entail? *(4 marks)*
c. How would you confirm the diagnosis of hepatocellular carcinoma (HCC)? *(2 marks)*
d. What are the criteria for liver transplantation in HCC? *(2 marks)*

8 *A 62-year-old woman presents to the accident and emergency department following trauma. A plain film of the tibia shows no fracture but reveals a focal lucency within the bone.*

a. What features do you need to assess? *(6 marks)*
b. The radiologist feels this may be a primary bone tumour. What should be done? *(4 marks)*

9 *A 43-year-old woman presents to her GP requesting a mammogram. She has no symptoms but is concerned after reading a newspaper article.*

a. What additional information do you need to provide advice? *(1 mark)*
b. Assuming these factors do not apply, what advice would you give? *(2 marks)*
c. What is the role of ultrasound and MRI? *(2 marks)*
d. Which patient groups are invited for breast cancer screening within the NHS? *(2 marks)*
e. In breast disease, what is meant by the term 'triple assessment' and when is this indicated? *(2 marks)*

10 *A previously healthy 52-year-old man undergoes a CT of the thorax following a road traffic accident. The only abnormality detected is a single 4-mm pulmonary nodule.*

a. What further information do you need before planning management? *(2 marks)*
b. What proportion of smokers will have a pulmonary nodule if screened? *(2 marks)*
c. Assuming the patient does smoke, what is the chance of this nodule being malignant? *(1 mark)*
d. What further investigations are indicated and which should be avoided at this stage? *(5 marks)*

MCQs answers

1. b. Abdominal ultrasound is the best first test looking for possible gallstones.
2. a. See Case 10.
3. d. The patient has a possible pulmonary embolus. V/Q is difficult to interpret in patients with cardiorespiratory disease.
4. c. The remainder result in lytic metastases.
5. e. The other lesions typically give ring enhancement.
6. e. The thalamus is a typical site of lacunar infarcts. The other features are classic signs of multiple sclerosis.
7. a. This is caused by infection with *Clostridium difficile*.
8. c.
9. d.
10. e. Diabetes mellitus is commonly seen in patients with cystic fibrosis.
11. a. Modern prostheses are MRI-compatible.
12. d. Triple assessment is used in symptomatic patients.
13. b.
14. d. Ultrasound has a low sensitivity for injuries to the solid abdominal viscera and CT should be performed.

15. a. Glass is usually radio-opaque.
16. a. See Case 23.
17. e. Pseudocysts take at least 4 weeks to develop.
18. e.
19. c.
20. b.
21. b. Myeloma does not show uptake of technetium compounds.
22. d. An unenhanced CT is the most sensitive investigation for renal calculi.
23. e. Rigler's sign is the ability to see both sides of the bowel wall and indicates a pneumoperitoneum.
24. b. See Case 11.
25. c. Less than this is stable disease. Progressive disease is an increase of 20%, or the presence of new lesions.
26. b. The other causes tend to give upper lobe fibrosis predominantly.
27. e. See Case 10.
28. a. Hepatic cysts have no blood supply.
29. c. Answers a, b and e are features of ulcerative colitis. Both ulcerative colitis and Crohn's disease predispose to oxalate urinary calculi.
30. c. Opiates cause aspiration pneumonia or pulmonary oedema.

Radiology: Clinical Cases Uncovered. By A. S. Shaw, E. M. Godfrey, A. Singh and T. F. Massoud. Published 2009 by Blackwell Publishing. ISBN 978-1-4051-8474-8.

PART 3: SELF-ASSESSMENT

EMQs answers

1
1. c
2. j
3. h
4. l
5. m

2
1. h
2. e
3. i
4. k
5. g

3
1. a
2. h
3. f
4. m
5. i

4
1. e
2. d
3. l
4. e
5. g

5
1. o
2. e
3. g
4. k
5. i

6
1. o
2. n
3. e
4. m
5. d

7
1. f
2. i
3. n
4. m
5. d

8
1. h
2. a
3. l
4. f
5. n

9
1. f
2. c
3. m
4. a
5. i

10
1. n
2. c
3. j
4. e
5. g

Radiology: Clinical Cases Uncovered. By A. S. Shaw, E. M. Godfrey,
A. Singh and T. F. Massoud. Published 2009 by Blackwell
Publishing. ISBN 978-1-4051-8474-8.

SAQs answers

1

a. Is there an associated headache (to suggest haemorrhage)? *(0.5 marks)* What was the time of onset (if potential for thrombolysis treatment)? *(0.5 marks)* Are there any predisposing factors in the past medical history (hypertension, known aneurysms)? *(1 mark)* What medication is the patient taking (espially anti-hypertensive agents and anticoagulants)? *(1 mark)*

b. CT scan of the head *(1 mark)*. Ideally, this should be combined with a post-contrast study either to look for perfusion defects in ischaemia or an aneurysm in cases of subarachnoid haemorrhage *(1 mark)*.

c. Initially, the blood pressure should be controlled medically *(1 mark)*. Definitive treatment may be achieved through endovascular *(1 mark)* or surgical techniques *(1 mark)*.

d. Endovascular therapy may result in damage to the arteries, including dissection or rupture, or extension of the area of infarction *(1 mark)*. Surgery may result in further haemorrhage or infarction *(1 mark)*. Each has its pros and cons and each case will need to be considered on its merits.

2

a. Deep vein thrombosis *(1 mark)* and venous obstruction by the pregnant uterus *(1 mark)*.

b. An ultrasound of deep veins of the right leg would look for a deep vein thrombosis *(1 mark)*. D-dimers would not be of any value as they are raised to 'abnormal' levels in pregnancy *(1 mark)*.

c. Pulmonary embolism *(1 mark)*.

d. The chest X-ray should be performed initially *(1 mark)* in order to look for other causes of breathlessness, particularly pneumothorax or

infection. A repeat ultrasound of both legs would avoid any radiation and may enable the diagnosis of thrombosis *(1 mark)*. If negative, the possibility of a pulmonary embolus can be investigated using either a ventilation–perfusion (V/Q) scan *(0.5 marks)* or CT pulmonary angiogram (CTPA) *(0.5 marks)* could be requested to look for pulmonary emboli. The V/Q scan exposes the mother to less radiation but the fetus to slightly more than a CTPA, *(1 mark)* but the CTPA is able to look for other causes of breathlessness *(1 mark)*.

3

a. Smoking history is crucial *(1 mark)*. Previous exposure to asbestos *(0.5 marks)* or an occupational history of exposure to dusts or other respiratory irritants *(0.5 marks)* may cause interstitial lung disease. Concomitant medical conditions, particularly connective tissue diseases *(1 mark)*, and medications are also potentially important *(1 mark)*.

b. A restrictive pattern with reduced total lung volume *(1 mark)*.

c. Bilateral pulmonary fibrosis *(1 mark)*, characterized by honeycomb pattern *(1 mark)* with a predominantly basal *(1 mark)* and subpleural *(1 mark)* distribution.

d. Usual interstitial pneumonitis, also known as cryptogenic fibrosing alveolitis or idiopathic pulmonary fibrosis *(1 mark)*.

4

a. No *(1 mark)*. In the absence of any 'red flag' signs, there is no indication for further X-rays *(1 mark)*.

b. 1 mSv is equivalent to 5 months background radiation *(1 mark)*.

c. Red flag signs: thoracic pain; fever; weight loss; bladder or bowel dysfunction; carcinoma history; neurological deficit; onset <20 years or >55 years *(Score 1 mark each, maximum 5 marks)*.

Radiology: Clinical Cases Uncovered. By A. S. Shaw, E. M. Godfrey, A. Singh and T. F. Massoud. Published 2009 by Blackwell Publishing. ISBN 978-1-4051-8474-8.

d. For neurological symptoms, an MRI *(1 mark)* would be best to examine just the spine. If systemic disease was suspected, a CT would be best *(1 mark)*.

5

a. CT colonography *(1 mark)*, CT abdomen and pelvis *(1 mark)* and barium enema *(1 mark)*.
b. CT colonography is the most accurate of the three, enabling detection of small polyps *(1 mark)* but requires 2 days of bowel preparation, air insufflation through a small rectal tube and intravenous hyoscine butylbromide *(1 mark)*.

   The conventional CT will only detect large tumours *(1 mark)* but requires only the drinking of oral contrast medium and intravenous contrast medium *(1 mark)*.

   The barium enema requires 2 days of bowel preparation *(1 mark)* but will only detect large polyps and frank tumours *(1 mark)*.
c. If the patient refuses colonoscopy, this should be clearly documented. A CT colonography is the next best test and should be performed on all but the most infirm patients unable to tolerate bowel preparation *(1 mark)*.

6

a. None. The diagnosis has been made *(1 mark)*.
b. Imaging (usually CT) is indicated to look for the complications of acute pancreatitis *(1 mark)*, most commonly necrosis and venous thrombosis *(0.5 marks each)*.
c. Gallstones, alcohol, drugs, anatomical variants, trauma, autoimmune disease *(0.5 marks each)*.
d. Ultrasound *(1 mark)* may be helpful in looking for gallbladder calculi *(1 mark)*. A magnetic resonance cholangiopancreatography (MRCP) study *(1 mark)* may be helpful to look for biliary abnormalities including anatomical variants of the ducts and ductal stones *(0.5 marks each)*.

7

a. To look for the complications of cirrhosis, principally the development of tumour *(0.5 marks)* and vascular abnormalities *(0.5 marks)*, either thrombosis or shunt vessels. This is achieved with 6-monthly ultrasound and serum α-fetoprotein (AFP) levels *(0.5 marks each)*.
b. This is a day-case procedure *(1 mark)*. The patient lies flat and local anaesthetic is injected in to the skin and down to the liver surface *(1 mark)*. The patient holds their breath and a biopsy needle is inserted in to the liver *(1 mark)*. Following the procedure there is a period of bed-rest, usually 6 hours, with regular observations *(1 mark)*. The major risk is bleeding, with approximately 1 in 1000 patients having a significant bleed *(1 mark)*. *(Maximum 4 marks)*
c. The lesion should have typical imaging features on two imaging modalities *(1 mark)*. Biopsy is controversial and is associated with an increased risk of tumour seeding *(1 mark)*.
d. One lesion up to 5 cm in diameter or up to three lesions each measuring less than 3 cm in diameter *(1 mark)* in the absence of extrahepatic disease *(1 mark)*.

8

a. The size and site (epiphysis, metaphysis, diaphysis) of the lesion *(1 mark each)*. Is the margin between the lesion and normal bone sharp or ill-defined? *(1 mark)* What density (calcification, lucent) is the matrix of the lesion? *(1 mark)* Is there a periosteal reaction? *(1 mark)* Is there a soft tissue component? *(1 mark)* Together with the patient's age, these will help to narrow down the differential diagnosis dramatically.

   Features suggestive of an aggressive lesion include an ill-defined margin, periosteal reaction and soft tissue extension.
b. Local staging with MRI, to include the whole of the affected bone *(1 mark)*. Assessment of the skeleton for other lesions with a bone scintigram *(1 mark)*. Systemic staging using CT *(1 mark)*. Biopsy should *not* be performed outside specialist referral units *(1 mark)*; the patient should be referred to such a unit urgently and this should not be delayed by awaiting the other investigations.

9

a. What is the patient's risk of developing breast cancer? *(1 mark)* This is primarily determined from the family history of breast cancer and the presence of any known genetic mutations.
b. The evidence for benefit of breast screening and risk from irradiating the breast tissue is much less clear in this age group. Mammography is less sensitive in dense *(1 mark)*, glandular breasts and the risk of inducing malignancy is higher *(1 mark)*. If the

patient insists, a further discussion at the local breast unit may help clarify this.

c. Ultrasound may be used as an adjunct in symptomatic patients or to guide biopsy of breast lesions *(1 mark)*. MRI is useful in screening young patients with high risk of developing breast cancer, where other imaging is equivocal and in those patients with breast implants *(1 mark)*.

d. Women aged 50–70 years at 3-yearly intervals *(1 mark)*. In the near future, this will change to 47–73 years. Women aged over 70 years may self-refer *(1 mark)*.

e. This is for symptomatic patients *(1 mark)*. It comprises clinical examination, mammography and ultrasound *(1 mark)*.

10

a. Does he smoke cigarettes? *(1 mark)* Does he have any other risk factors for lung cancer? *(1 mark)*

b. Approximately 50% of smokers will have a pulmonary nodule *(1 mark)*. On successive screening rounds, 10% of patients will develop a new nodule *(1 mark)*.

c. Approximately 1% *(1 mark)*.

d. The recommendations of the Fleischner Society are for a follow-up CT in 6–12 months and then 18–24 months if no change *(2 marks)*. The lesion is too small for a positron emission tomography (PET) study *(1 mark)* or percutaneous biopsy *(1 mark)*. The balance of risk does not justify an open biopsy *(1 mark)*.

Index of cases by diagnosis

Index

Note: page numbers in *italics* refer to figures, those in **bold** refer to tables and boxes